RESETTLEMENT FROM LARGE PSYCHIATRIC HOSPITAL TO SMALL COMMUNITY RESIDENCE

For Thomas, Jean, Andrea and Rebecca

Resettlement from Large Psychiatric Hospital to Small Community Residence

One Step to Freedom?

R. V. E. FORRESTER-JONES
GORDON GRANT
Centre for Social Policy Research and Development
University of Wales
Bangor
Gwynedd

Avebury
Aldershot · Brookfield USA · Hong Kong · Singapore · Sydney

Published by
Avebury
Ashgate Publishing Ltd
Gower House
Croft Road
Aldershot
Hants GU11 3HR
England

Ashgate Publishing Company
Old Post Road
Brookfield
Vermont 05036
USA

British Library Cataloguing in Publication Data

Forrester-Jones, R. V. E.
Resettlement from large psychiatric hospital to small community residence : one step to freedom?. - (Studies in care in the community)
1. Mentally ill - Social networks - Great Britain 2. Mentally ill - Rehabilitation Great Britain 3. Mentally ill - Housing - Great Britain 4. Mentally ill - Government policy - Great Britain
I. Title II. Grant, Gordon
362.2 '23' 0941 [F}

ISBN 1 85972 363 2

Library of Congress Catalog Card Number: 96-79375

Printed in Great Britain by
Antony Rowe Ltd, Chippenham, Wiltshire

Contents

Figures and tables

Acknowledgements

The authors owe a particular debt of gratitude to twenty-five people who, as residents of new community housing projects, allowed us access to their everyday life experiences following resettlement from a psychiatric hospital. They demonstrated that warmth, affection and hope can surface when interest precedes. Anonymity prevents us from thanking them more personally. The research would not have been possible without the co-operation and help of managers and staff at the hospital and at the two community housing projects. We acknowledge your patience and forbearance. Special thanks are due to Dr Charles Crosby and members of the Health Services Research Unit at the University of Wales Bangor for their helpful advice and preparedness to share data and experiences. None of this endeavour would have come to fruition without the help of three colleagues: Brian Jones for his artistry and technical expertise in conjuring the diagrams in the text, Emma Howard for the painstaking and largely unrewarding task of proof-reading, and finally Sue Howard for re-typing the text more times than we can remember, and each time with customary skill and unfailing humour. Finally, we acknowledge the ESRC for a competition studentship grant which funded the research.

You feel much better being out of hospital. You feel like you are chained up and when you go out you are free, free as a bird.

Robert

Introduction

Genesis, policy context and guide to study

> ...everyone needs a network of people from whom to receive and to whom to give support.
>
> (Turner-Crowson, 1993)

We may all remember situations within our personal histories where we can trace people who have supported us, or times when such help has been missing in our lives. Personal experience will probably tell most of us that we do indeed need supportive relationships which help to give us a sense of belonging, security, identity and well-being.

The people whose lives and relationships are documented in this work belong to a group of persons who have been characterised as generally reserved, have a tendency to enjoy youthful good looks which belie their chronological age (Howe, 1995, p.102) and include some of the most creative, talented individuals such as Beethoven, William Blake, Samuel Coleridge, Leonardo da Vinci, Herman Melville, Sylvia Plath and Virginia Woolf (Lefley, 1996, p.3). Membership of such a group lies in a diagnosis of having mental health problems. The 25 people who are the focus of this study have all been diagnosed at some point in their lives as having psychiatric illnesses, and they have all spent long periods of time in large Victorian mental hospitals. They are now living in the community. Given the appropriate medication and adequate social support, most people with psychiatric problems (approximately one person in every hundred) can lead normal lives in the community (Meise and Fleischhacker, 1996). However, Jones (1995) argues that in the present state of research 'we know much more about medication than we do about the kinds of social support they need'. This book is written as a modest contribution towards redressing this imbalance.

Social networks for people with mental health problems as a topic for research was suggested by the second author (GG) who has a long standing research interest in the dynamics of informal support and in the development of frameworks for assessing the needs of informal carers. The idea was developed further by the first author (RF-J) with the aid of an ESRC competition studentship grant for a PhD thesis.

The study locations of two market towns in rural Wales were for the first author familiar since she had been brought up and educated in the area. Castleton Hospital was frosted in her memory as a large ornate Victorian building set in expansive grounds including every facility, surrounded by rural countryside. However, as a result of the White Paper, Caring for People (DoH, 1989) and the NHS and Community Care Act (1990) which laid the foundations for a reorganised mixed economy approach to community care, this hospital was now due for closure and with it the resettlement of people for whom the institution had been home for so long. Immediate questions sprang to mind about who would support, befriend and show affection towards these individuals and how they might be able to adapt to a new life within the local community.

The White Paper restated government commitment to:

> a new style of service (which) offers a much higher quality of life for people with a mental illness and a service more appreciated by their families than is possible in the traditional large and often remote mental hospital. The Government reaffirms its support of the policy as a civilised and humanitarian one (para 7.4).

Following the White Paper, the Protocol for Investment in Health Gain - Mental Health (Welsh Office, 1993) gave a clear message about reappraising people's needs and circumstances holistically. Policy was also directed towards enabling far more people to be treated from a permanent home base, rather than being confined to a long-stay hospital, as the following health gain target in the Protocol suggests:

> (to) increase the proportion of those with a severe mental illness who have a permanent home with appropriate levels of support to 75 per cent by 1997, and to 90 per cent by 2002 (p.9)

Strategic goals at the core of the protocol were directed towards: reducing the number of premature deaths associated with mental health problems, improving quality of life, reducing the impact of socio-economic factors on mental distress and relapse associated with mental illness, and reducing stigma attached to mental health problems (p.8). The protocol also set a target for 1994 for the development of comprehensive information packs for users and also for the development of methods for assessing quality of life. Care assessment and diagnostic and social disability reviews built into individual care plans and individual planning were seen as fundamental to maximising the effectiveness of the rehabilitation process.

Care in the community as a more appropriate alternative to hospital care for people with mental health problems has been advocated in government documents since the 1950s (Ham, 1992). Factors culminating in the deinstitution movement have been mulled over and mirror those in the USA (Turner-Crowson, 1993). They are multifarious and include firstly the 'scientific innovation' of drug treatment beginning in the 1950s. The psychotropic drug revolution made it possible to treat the symptoms of many mental disorders cheaply outside of hospital (Roberts, 1967; Jones, 1988; Taylor and Taylor, 1989; Healy, 1991; Bury, 1992; Prior, 1993; Cotterill, 1994; Meise and Fleischhacker, 1996). Developing concurrently with medication for the mentally ill were sociological and psychological theories which suggested that mental illness was less a disease and more a reaction to societal living (Jenner et al. 1993). Harmonising with these theories was 'societal reactionism' to labelling and stereotyping people as mentally ill (Lemert, 1951; Becker, 1963; Goffman, 1961; Rosenhan, 1973; Taylor, 1994/5).

The classic work of 'Asylums' by Goffman (1961) was perhaps the main force behind the emerging 'anti-institutionalism' which critiqued hospital and traditional psychiatric practices as oppressive and institutionalising (Foucault, 1961; Barton, 1959; Szasz, 1961, 1971, 1973; Faber, 1993) and called instead for individualised non stigmatising therapeutic approaches to care (Solomon and Marcenko, 1992). This was coupled with growing public concern over deteriorating conditions, neglect and harsh treatment experienced by patients of large long-stay hospitals and nursing homes (Belknap, 1956; Caudhill, 1958; Dunham and Weinberg, 1960; Robb, 1967; King et al. 1971; Martin, 1984; Geller and Harris, 1994) which was vividly portrayed in novels such as Ken Kesey's One Flew Over the Cuckoo's Nest (1962).

Another argument within the discourse about changes in mental health care is 'psychiatric determinism' (Prior, 1993) which refers to changes in knowledge, organisation and management treatment and care from within the psychiatric system.

Many research reports indicated the benefits and cost-effectiveness of treating and supporting people in their own homes and communities (Knapp et al. 1992, 1994). Accompanying value shifts represented best by the normalisation philosophy and later social role valorisation (SRV) (Nirje, 1969; Wolfensberger, 1983) which emphasised the idea that conditions of everyday living which are 'as close as possible to the regular circumstances and ways of life of society' should be made available to people with disabilities (Nirje, 1969) became more widespread. Legal and judicial pressures to protect patients' rights, emphasising use of non restrictive forms of care (Brown, 1985), added weight to normalisation principles.

Economic necessity or a belief that fiscal problems in the economy would be lessened by an alternative cheaper form of care in the community rather than maintaining expensive large mental hospitals is perhaps the argument used most strongly and negatively by the media and others (Walker, 1982; Scull, 1984; Jones, 1988; Turner-Crowson, 1993). The closure of hospitals would release capital and, potentially at least, create revenue savings, reducing direct costs to the National Health Service (Korman and Glennerster, 1990). This was paralleled by New Right ideology suggesting that pluralistic forms of service provision leads to efficiency and effectiveness for the economy and for service users (Cahill, 1994; Taylor, 1994/5).

Whatever the real underpinnings of the new community care policies, lessons from the past have nevertheless introduced a cautionary note into hospital closure. Policy and Ministerial approval for closure under the new procedures will not be granted unless it can be demonstrated that adequate community-based alternatives have been developed, particularly for those who have spent many years in long-stay hospitals (Audit Commission, 1994). Media attention on unfortunate incidents where community care has failed both its recipients (Ritchie et al. 1994; McNeice, 1996) and other victims (the Zito tragedy in 1992) has led to a number of initiatives by government to improve present problems such as the lack of coordination between social services and NHS Trusts (Department of Health, 1995). The Health Secretary, Stephen Dorrell, has also been reported as having recently announced a fund of over £95 million to expand community care services, and a Patients Charter on Mental Health specifying the services that those with mental health problems have the right to expect from the NHS at national and at a local level (Brindle, 1996). Furthermore, the Mental Health (Patients in the Community) Act (1995) aims to 'ensure more effective, care and supervision for people with severe mental illness' (Department of Health, 1996, p.1). Specialist care will be based on the Care Programme Approach under which everyone with mental health problems living in the community will have an after-care plan and a 'supervisor' (key worker).

As will become apparent there are still significant ambiguities about the meaning of community care for it can be argued that it has become something of a slogan to justify the means to reach potentially quite different politically motivated ends (Bulmer, 1987). The closure of the great Victorian asylums was anticipated over three decades ago as representing a formidable organisational task by no less a person than the then Minister of Health (Powell, 1961). The power of resistance to change which Enoch Powell predicted so well has since given way to a more liberal approach which relies on enlisting the interests of the community, as well as the winning over of the traditionalist psychiatric establishment. But what kind of community are we now releasing people into? What are the essential features of the new 'homely' environments into which people with long-term mental health problems are being placed? How do people adapt to a new life in the community after many years spent in hospital? How do individuals construe their personal and social lives in different community settings, and the support they receive? And to what extent can people be said to be a part of the community as well as just in it?

These are not idle questions. Indeed, despite the cumulative and colourful history of institutional care, of the rush to empty long-stay hospitals in the 1960s and 1970s, of the rhetoric about the desirability of community care, there is still thought to be a scarcity of studies which have considered the benefits to individuals of different types of community housing (Huxley et al. 1990; Howe, 1995). Moreover, accounts which are based within the everyday experiences of residents are all the more rare. Hence, despite the steady accumulation of knowledge about deinstitutionalisation the voice of the service user has been none too evident.

Present policy rhetoric is couched in terms such as 'choice' and 'independence'. Indeed, these are key watchwords in the White Paper itself: 'Promoting choice and independence underlie all the Government's proposals' (DoH, 1989). According to the White Paper (para 1.8) the attendant policy changes are intended to:

> enable people to live as normal a life as possible in their own homes or in a homely environment in the community; provide the right amount of care and support to help people achieve maximum possible independence and, by acquiring or reacquiring basic living skills, help them to achieve their full potential; give people a greater individual say in how they live their lives and the services they need to help them do so.

This more individualised approach to supporting people inclines towards a model which is bent on listening to, and being prepared to act on, what those who use services have to say, though critics question whether the necessary resources will be made available and whether there is the basis of a community left which can care (Langan, 1991). Psychiatric hospital resettlement and hospital closure is thus taking place in a highly charged political arena. However, this means that research which can begin to capture the experiences of those at the receiving end is of increased significance.

Briefly stated, this was the prevailing policy context at the time the present research took place. However, it is necessary to say something about the research parameters which informed the approach to the study.

Studies in a variety of service and cultural contexts have begun to show the value of conditioning factors in people's lives through social network analysis (for example, Pattison et al. 1979; d'Abbs, 1982; Greenblatt et al. 1982; Wenger, 1984; House et al. 1988; Cutrona and Suhr, 1994; Ell, 1996) and that access to support or information, personal health, adaptation in old age, stress reduction and coping can all be linked to the structure and functioning of social networks, and whether those networks serve to provide individuals with support commensurate with needs. It was also anticipated, as people with long-term mental health problems were moved from hospital to community, that a social network approach would help to throw some light on the potential for assisting individuals towards living a more socially integrated life in the community. Specifically an applied social network analysis was seen as a convenient method for gathering data about the structure of individuals' social networks, the strength of ties within them, and the functions these appear to serve for individuals, including relationships with community members. However, how individuals with mental health problems necessarily construe the contacts and support that may be available to them through their networks is another matter, and something thought to be studied best through ethnography.

The adopted research approach was therefore one which combined applied social network analysis with ethnography although, as will be seen in later chapters, use was made of other methods too. Brought together the two underlying approaches can be seen as a form of pluralistic evaluation (Smith and Cantley, 1985).

The study can be viewed on four levels: firstly, as an attempt to test and extend knowledge about the concept of social networks and how they may serve to mediate the adjustment of individuals; secondly, to add to the apparently scarce accounts of mental health services from the perspective of those who use them; thirdly, to consider whether local community housing projects provide the kind of contexts for the living out of everyday lives which are in line with intended policy, and; finally, to provide some pointers which may help purchasers and providers of services to offer people forms of individualised support which they need or want.

At the local level, a rural Wales health authority had sought to mirror aforementioned policy ideals by the gradual but systematic closure of wards in the large Victorian hospital at Castleton and in a sister hospital, at Small Market, a nearby town, with the transfer of residents to community settings in the county. The sister hospital was the first to close down its wards and, at the start of this study, 15 residents had already moved to a project called Greentrees set up by the local health authority in 1989. Ten individuals from three rehabilitation wards in Castleton hospital had also been relocated into Mountain View, a large house consisting of three single and three shared flats.

A comparative evaluation of institutional and community mental health services was already in process when the present study began. Conducted by the Health Services Research Unit (HSRU) at the University of Wales Bangor, this involved a large-scale longitudinal study of individuals' psychiatric state, behaviour and quality of life. An interim report (Barry et al. 1990, p.89) had already indicated that:

> Social relations [are] an important aspect of residents' lives and have important implications about how residents will adjust to and cope with life in the community.

The present study was aimed at further exploration of the significance of the social context of residents' lives at a time of transition. This was to be conducted by means of a qualitative in-depth study of two community housing projects in Small Market and Castleton to which 25 long-stay hospital residents had been discharged.

The HSRU research had been commissioned by a consortium of agencies and was primarily geared to evaluate the effectiveness of the hospital closure programme and its effects on residents. By contrast, this complementary study provided an opportunity to spend a considerable period of time in the field, living, working and associating with residents as they lived out their daily lives. However, a fruitful relationship was forged with the HSRU team which gave the researchers access not only to pertinent research data which helped to inform their own study but also to a group of colleagues whose intellectual stimulation and advice was invaluable.

The primary aims of the research were as follows:

1 to describe the structure of the social networks of previously hospitalised long-stay psychiatric residents now living in the community;

2 to assess the importance of networks of relationships to individuals and the potential importance of those relationships to the social integration of individuals in the community;

3 to explore the philosophy and care practices in two dissimilar community housing projects, Greentrees and Mountain View, with a view to gauging how these mediated residents' experience of life in the community.

There was an opportunity to engage in a short follow up study five years after the initial research had begun. Changes experienced by both projects and in the social care and lives of the individuals in this study are therefore provided.

In Chapter 1 social network and social support concepts are introduced and different methodological approaches to an assessment of network structure and functioning are reviewed. Parameters of networks are described and an attempt is made to assess, from the literature, the connections between social networks, social support, mental health, social functioning and social integration.

A chronologically based account of how the study was conceptualised and implemented is given in Chapter 2. An argument is made for a multi-method approach which in this case involved an applied social network analysis with ethnography.

The two community housing projects, their aims, philosophy, staffing and resources in relation to local mental health policy are described in Chapter 3 and biographical, psychiatric and behavioural details of residents are also provided. In Chapter 4 the results of an applied social network analysis are presented. These give some insights into the structure of individuals' social networks, individual variation, and contrasts between residents living in the two separate community housing schemes.

A house by house description of care practices is presented in Chapter 5 with an attempt to unpack and explain the factors that have come to influence them. The account is based in the working experiences of the staff by means of observation and participation in the self same practices. The findings point to the existence of several 'models' of care. The implications of the practices for the development of individuals' social networks are considered.

Vignettes of residents are given in Chapter 6 to provide insight and understanding of the lives of people with mental health problems. This forms the basis for subsequent analyses in Chapters 7, 8 and 9. A re-evaluation of data pertaining to structural properties of networks (Chapter 4) using case study analysis indicates that qualitative methods provide more reliable accounts of the social lives of individuals with a mental illness.

Following the case study vignettes dimensions of support based on the findings are introduced in Chapter 7 and an attempt is made to assess how these are experienced by residents in the two housing schemes

How residents view their relationships with network members is the focus of Chapter 8. In particular the conflicts and contradictions in maintaining old or familiar ties are illustrated for these are seen to provide continuity and meaning at a time of change and transition in people's lives. On the other hand, the potential for making new ties in the community and the benefits that may come from them are also illustrated.

In Chapter 9 the results of how social networks and social support mediate individuals' mental health, social functioning and social integration are discussed.

Summary and conclusions regarding theory building about social networks, community care policy and mental health practice are given in Chapter 10. Suggestions for further research are put forward.

Names of individuals, agencies and places have been anonymised throughout the text.

1 Social networks, social support and well-being

> The distribution of supportive ties and behavior throughout a network influences the ways that the social architecture of life is qualitatively experienced and interpreted by community members.
>
> (Albrecht, 1994)

Introduction

In a recent review of the contribution of medical sociology to the study of severe mental illness Cook and Wright (1995) draw attention to the need for more research into the effects of stigma, community integration and networks, consumer and family movements, social control and finally client outcomes. Two of these themes in particular are highly relevant to the concerns of this chapter. Regarding community integration and networks, they emphasise the importance of being able to view the social environments of people with psychiatric disabilities in more dynamic ways, particularly the interactional processes of reciprocal support and strain. They stress the need for continued exploration of the structure and function of people's social networks and how these contextual factors shape service utilisation and outcomes. On the subject of client outcomes they point to shifts in interest and emphasis from clinical to behavioural and quality of life outcomes. What is especially salient, however, is the emphasis Cook and Wright place on bringing together different 'tributaries' of interest. Drawing on Pearlin (1992) they suggest that questions for 'structure seekers' (those interested in the consequences of social structure for health) and 'meaning seekers' (those who study the effects of social meaning on health) need to be brought together: 'it is in the "creative integration" of these different perspectives in medical sociology that the answers to the most pressing questions and problems can be found' (Cook and Wright, 1995, p.107).

In this chapter an attempt is made to review literature about social networks and social support and to tie that knowledge to outcome considerations, about how people adapt to life in the community following long-term hospitalisation. However, following Cook and Wright's (1995) propositions we attempt to draw on both quantitative and more recent qualitative research in order to link structural and interpretive issues in the everyday experiences of people with severe mental illness. Initially it is necessary to discuss the related, though often confused, concepts of social networks and social support.

The concept of the social network

A universally accepted definition of the term 'social network' is impossible to establish as writers have tended to emphasise different definitional criteria applicable to specific contexts. Barnes (1954) suggests that social network refers to a web of relationships attached to an individual whilst Mitchell (1969, p.2) defines social network as a specific set of linkages among a defined set of persons.

These definitions present a structural approach to the understanding of social networks. Network studies have tended to concentrate on the structural properties of networks like size, density, membership and linkages perhaps because these are the most amenable for study. Latterly there has been more interest in the function or content of relationships embedded within networks. The function or content of relationships within a network has been described as the most important item of information about it as it indicates something of the goods and services exchanged, the closeness or intimacy between members, the intensity of their interactions and the exchange of information involved (Bulmer, 1987).

All of these 'functions' may be regarded as potentially supportive features of the social network although the literature has tended to be unclear in its terminology. The social network may therefore be regarded as an opportunity framework of relationships which may or may not provide social support. In this respect, the presence of a social relationship is a necessary precondition for the provision of social support. The literature suggests that the structural properties of social networks have attracted considerable attention from researchers whilst the functions and content of social support have been rather less in evidence, perhaps because they are more difficult to conceptualise and measure.

Quantitative social network studies

Quantitative analyses of social networks have usually dealt with the structural properties of the social network, that is, those properties which give the social network its 'shape', so presenting what could be termed an 'opportunity structure' for meeting the needs of individuals. Thus, for example, studies emphasise the *size*, or number of people constituting a network (Weiss, 1974; Hammer et al. 1978;

Sokolovsky and Cohen, 1981; Leff et al. 1990). *Density*, which refers to the ratio of people in a network known to each other, has not been so frequently studied (Tolsdorf, 1976; Taylor et al. 1984). *Anchorage* and *reachability* have been construed respectively as the length of pathways to others from specific individuals, and the extent to which individuals can contact and use people important to them without going through too many steps (Mitchell, 1969). Together with size, *membership* is perhaps the other most commonly measured trait in network structures, though there has perhaps been a tendency to oversimplify membership categories, viz. 'family', 'friends', 'professional supporters', so clouding important issues about normative expectations for mutual support and power relationships. There is the issue of the *homogeneity* of network members in terms of their similarity or dissimilarity of age, gender, race, ethnicity, religiosity and so on though, with perhaps the exception of age and gender, such parameters have been rarely reported (d'Abbs, 1982). Finally, studies have also very commonly reported the *frequency* of interaction between individuals (Rosser and Harris, 1965; Wenger, 1984; Dunn et al. 1990 amongst many others).

Studies which emphasise network structure, perhaps at the expense of considerations about the function and content of relationships, have led to assumptions as to what is the 'right' network structure for a given type of support. Weiss (1974) and Henderson (1977) argue, for example, that different types of support come from different relationships within the social network. This leads one to conclude that it is not only the structure of the social network that is important in providing a possible *context* for support, but rather the nature of the supporting behaviour itself and how this is construed by those involved. This is supported by Walker et al. (1977) who contend that the type of support provided to individuals depends on the structure of the social network and also the quality of support provided by the relationships.

The aforementioned studies have tended to rely upon interviewing and the ability of the interviewee to name people in their network. It might be argued that, as informants, individuals with mental health problems may not wish to or be able to answer in this way. This was certainly found to be a problem in the more recent study by Dunn et al. (1990). Relying very much as they do on interviewing, these studies make heavy demands on the ability of people to communicate as well as to recall persons in their networks. Dunn et al. (1990) in their observational study found that communication between psychiatric patients was in the main non-verbal, suggesting that there is likely to be a need for studies which deploy a range of data collection strategies.

Quantitative studies have also been applied to the more qualitative dimensions of networks and have tended to concentrate more on the interactions involved in relationships and their supportiveness. These refer to their emotional valence, for example whether the behaviours are supportive or destructive; warm, friendly, intimate, confidential; tolerant, cheering, comforting; or the opposite, and so on (Greenblatt et al. 1982; Dufåker, 1994). Studies have considered the *content* of relationships in terms of the nature of functions or the meanings individuals give to these functions (Wenger, 1984; Litwak and Szelenyi, 1969). Some studies have laid a stress on the *directedness* within relationships, that is the amount of reciprocity between members or the direction of interaction and involvement (Mitchell, 1969; Grant, 1993). *Intensity* has been described as referring to the strength of commitment between individuals, or alternatively the intimacy which is felt (Brown and Harris, 1978; Dunn et al. 1990).

However, as already stated, such studies tell us little about what social networks mean to individuals. Qualitative studies have attempted to gain subjective as well as objective data but again have tended to rely on self-report questionnaires based on large-scale survey approaches (Lehman, 1980; Barrera, 1978). The danger with attempts to quantify or objectify social networks and social support in these ways is that it too easily leads to the notion of networks having an existence of their own independent of the social constructions and understandings that individual network members bring to the situation.

The concept of social support

'Social support' has proved an elusive concept and there appears not to be any general or uniting theory as to what social support is or what its place is within social network theory. For example some researchers have argued that the social support system exists within the social network (Caplan, 1974), this being analogous to the relational content of interpersonal ties described by House et al. (1988). However, others have suggested that the social support system may be synonymous with the social network and have used the terms interchangeably, as for example Greenblatt et al. (1982). This lack of a specific theoretical framework (Ell, 1996) has led to a certain degree of confusion. Others have used different terminology to understand the difference between social networks and social support systems, for example, primary and secondary networks and personal and general networks e.g. Collins and Pancoast (1976). However, Hammer (1981, p.45) states:

> The difference between social networks and support systems is not a mere terminological distinction, since it leads to different formulations of the research problems, with different choices of the kinds of measures to be used, different perspectives on the role of basic social research, and a different potential for theoretical analysis.

With these contentions of terminology, what then are we to make of the term? The literature has provided some typologies of social support which are worthy of consideration at this point. Support typologies are a good way of systematising data and have been used extensively by anthropologists and sociologists to understand social phenomena such as ageing (Wenger, 1992), community (Collins and Pancoast, 1976) and mental well-being (Gottlieb, 1983).

Many different classification schemes have been developed for distinguishing between different types of support. These have varied from the basic and broad ranging to the more specific and have been either derived empirically or drawn from the theoretical literature. At the broadest level is the dual typology of Pattison (1977) who identified two types of support: instrumental (tangible forms of support such as personal care, financial assistance, goods, services and information (Kropotkin, 1914; Wirth, 1938; Willmott and Young, 1962; Anderson, 1971; Laslett, 1972)) and affective (emotional, social reinforcement, recognition and esteem building, (Brown and Harris, 1978; Kahn and Antonucci, 1980; House, 1981)).

As research has progressed, more detailed taxonomies have been developed. Gottlieb's (1978) typology draws empirically from the descriptions of informal helping behaviours of single mothers. The typology identified emotionally supportive behaviours, problem-solving behaviours, indirect personal influence and environmental action. Gottlieb found that different types of support were provided for different problems. The mothers in his study reported that they received emotional support for emotional problems, emotional and problem-solving support for problems related to their children, and problem-solving support for financial problems.

Kahn and Antonucci (1980), again collecting data on how 'ordinary' people see support, have defined social support using the three 'A's. These are namely affect (caring and emotional intimacy); affirmation (provision of information about the rightness or wrongness of one's action or thoughts) and aid (direct help through money, time and effort).

House (1981) identifies four types of support behaviours in connection with 'work stress'. These are emotional support (esteem, affect, trust, concern, listening), appraisal support (affirmation, feedback, social comparison), informational support (advice, suggestion, directives, information); and instrumental support (aid in kind, money, labour, time, modifying environment) (House, 1981, p.23).

Barrera and Ainlay (1983) include six categories of social support drawn from a content analysis of reviewed research articles. These are material aid (providing tangible materials such as financial help); behavioural assistance (sharing of tasks); intimate interaction (counselling behaviours such as listening, caring and understanding); guidance (offering advice, information or instruction); feedback (providing individuals with feedback about their behaviours, thoughts or feelings); positive social interaction (engaging in social interactions for fun and/or relaxation).

The strength of this particular typology lies within the descriptions in each category which identify the behaviours associated with each type of support (Vaux, 1988).

In her longitudinal study of changing help in old age, Wenger (1992) identifies three types of social support: emotional support; routine household chores and household maintenance; and personal care.

More recently, Richman et al. (1993) have identified eight forms of social support, again from a content analysis on the literature of both ill and well individuals, based on a practice model developed for clinical use. The eight types of support are namely (a) listening (Gottlieb, 1983; Sarason et al. 1983); (b) emotional (Caplan et al. 1980; Veiel et al. 1991) (c) emotional challenge (Plas et al. 1985) (d) reality confirmation (Gottlieb, 1983; Kahn and Antonucci, 1980) (e) task appreciation (House, 1981), (f) task challenge (Sarason et al. 1983), (g) tangible assistance (Cobb, 1979; House, 1981) and (h) personal assistance (House, 1981; Kahn and Antonucci, 1980 and Wellman, 1985).

Finally Bowers (1987), although referring primarily to caregiving, argues that most of the recent empirical work has so far adopted task-based definitions. She contends that much of the work of caring is invisible and therefore has tended to have been overlooked. Bowers argues that many of the components of caring are deliberately kept invisible from dependants in order to preserve their self-esteem and sense of autonomy. Working from a grounded theory approach, Bowers constructed a typology of care including anticipatory care (based on anticipated future need), preventive care (monitoring at a distance residents' medication, diets and so forth), supervisory care (direct intervention such as assistance with taking medication) and instrumental care (actually 'doing for' residents). Underpinning this was protective care whose purpose was to maintain the self-esteem of the dependent. This involves minimising their awareness of their failing abilities and maximising the extent to which they still perceive themselves as independent (Nolan and Grant, 1992). Bowers' (1987) model, based on a sample of children caring for parents suffering from dementia, was intended as an exploratory rather than an explanatory model. Like some of the other typologies or taxonomies, the categories she uses are not all mutually exclusive. These have recently been extended by Nolan et al. (1995).

What emerges from the above is that the literature tends to focus on 'social support' as an independent or conditioning variable that 'functions' to aid an individual's health and personal well-being (Kaplan et al. 1977; Eurelings-Bontekoe et al. 1995). It is argued that this idea of social support aiding mental health has its roots in the classical sociological traditions, such as Durkheim's (1952) theory of social integration and its relationship to suicide rates. It also stems from other classical sociological traditions in which it is theorised that all humans have needs which can only be met through social interaction with others.

Thus, social support may function as a preventive agent of physical or mental disease. However, while many researchers have speculated about the importance of social support in the aetiology, precipitation, course of and recovery from disease, Kaplan et al. (1977) argue that there is little strong empirical evidence to confirm this importance. They state that this is due to the fact that attempts at conceptualisation and measurement have been inadequate and discipline-bound.

Studies show that support provided by informal carers can prove to be a highly variable commodity in terms of its availability, scope, stability and adaptability for people disadvantaged in different ways (Berkowitz, 1986; Vaughn and Leff, 1976; Grant and Wenger, 1993). There is also evidence to suggest that not all support, whether provided by formal or informal means, is necessarily construed by recipients as being helpful, either because it is not needed, more or less than needed, or engenders a false sense of self-efficacy (Rook, 1992). Furthermore, Eurelings-Bontekoe et al. (1995) argue that from a clinical perspective the adverse aspects of social support need as much attention as the positive ones.

Similarly Ell (1996) has offered a critique of literature on social support which, she asserts, has overemphasised its beneficial effects. She suggests that an individual's recovery or adaptation following chronic illness is assumed to be negatively affected when family support is absent. Rather, she argues that those who seek to support others can consciously or unconsciously provoke stress and that negative social exchanges can and do occur between network members.

More recently it has been argued that it is much less clear what it is about social relationships, and social support, that affects health and well-being and how this is occasioned. House et al. (1988) contend that three aspects of social relationships - their existence and quantity, their formal structure, and their functional content - must be conceptually and empirically distinguished. These were termed social integration, social networks and relational content respectively. The concept of social support is one type of relational content, the others being suggested as (i) relational demands and conflicts and (ii) social regulation or control. Social integration and networks can be seen as representing structures of social relationships that affect health and well-being while social support, relational demands and regulation are social processes through which these structures have their effects. This conceptualisation is central to the present study which uses ideas about both the structure of social networks and the supportive content of those networks as a means of understanding how individuals' social lives are constituted and interpreted by individuals with long-term mental health problems.

An interesting contribution to this continuing debate comes from Murrell et al.'s (1992) study of older adults. Two dimensions of social support were measured: a functional measure termed 'anticipated help' and a structural measure of the strength of the social networks termed 'social integration'. The study was also of note in that it concentrated on the impacts of positive affect rather than distress or ill health of subjects. Functional and structural support both contributed to happiness in older adults, but in different ways. Functional support appeared to have an enduring positive relationship to positive affect but neither influenced nor was influenced by events. By contrast, structural support did not have enduring direct effects on positive affect but did influence and was itself influenced by events. To quote the authors:

> The feeling of security based on perceived support availability may be needed to maintain positive affect over time and the opportunity for sharing on the basis of social integration may be important for gaining the psychological benefits of desirable events but may not be sufficient in itself for maintaining positive affect beyond six months or so.
>
> (Murrell et al. 1992, p.568)

The authors go on to hypothesise that it is the feeling of accomplishment derived from meeting challenging events that is the critical feature to hold in mind here, and that 'promoting' experiences that give older adults even a modest sense of accomplishment would seem to have potential as a target for effective mental health intervention (ibid, p.569).

Social support, social networks and mental health

Previous research has shown that the social environment and in particular social relationships play a significant role in mediating mental health (Eisemann and Perris, 1985; Pattison, 1977; Cohen and Sokolovsky, 1978a; Hammer et al. 1978; Sokolovsky et al. 1978; Cohen and Sokolovsky, 1979). In this respect social networks can act, or function, as social support systems to promote mental health. The social support system may be crudely defined as a group of connections formed with persons that are likely to be seen often, that are regarded as intimates, and with whom emotional, physical, economic and informational support are exchanged (Greenblatt et al. 1982). A social support system may therefore be merely a part of, or synonymous with, a wider personal social network.

Studies of social networks of 'well' people have tended to emphasise physical, economic, emotional and social support functions (for example, Wirth, 1938; Barnes, 1954; Mitchell, 1969), and have linked these to the operation of exchange relationships. However, when one of the parties to a potential exchange relationship develops a chronic illness or disability the possibility of maintaining reciprocities within ties may become problematic, and even the maintenance of ties may become difficult. In this connection the literature suggests three main hypotheses about the mediating relationship between social support and mental health.

The first hypothesis concerns the idea that a lack of social relationships is implicated in the development of neurotic disorders independent of adversity. This hypothesis has been advocated in studies by Henderson et al. (1980) and Lin et al. (1979). Many subsequent studies have also produced evidence that the lack of social support is associated with increased morbidity (Pearlin et al. 1981; Holahan and Moos, 1981; Aneshensel and Stone, 1982; Aneshensel and Frerichs, 1982). The influence behind such a hypothesis can be traced to Bowlby's study in which he identified social causes (in Bowlby's case maternal deprivation) of neurosis (Bowlby, 1969, 1973, 1980) (Henderson et al. 1980, p.723). However, Henderson's (1980) longitudinal study of a general population sample failed to confirm the hypothesis. His Interview Schedule For Social Interaction (ISSI) which systematically examines an individual's personal network and his/her satisfaction with it found that it was not the individual's social environment that was important in the prevention of neurosis, but how the individual construes it (Henderson, 1985, p.48). This points to the importance of understanding people's social constructions of their lives and their living environments and how these are appraised, rather than relying merely on independent objective assessments or the researcher's own assessments.

The second hypothesis it that social support is a stress-buffer (Cassel, 1976) in that it acts as a cushion against the impact of life stresses, thereby reducing morbidity. This has been developed in many studies (Antonovsky, 1974; Cobb, 1976; Henderson, 1977; Brown and Harris, 1978), and has its roots in the growing scientific and clinical conviction that stress and life changes may be a significant factor in a wide variety of psychiatric and physical disorders (Lin and Dean, 1985, p.123). It may be anticipated that the disruptive and potentially stressful effects of relocation from hospital to community might be mediated by the existence of supportive ties. A key to understanding the processes involved is likely to be the degree to which 'official' definitions of support are in harmony with those constructions of supportiveness which residents bring to the situation. Other, perhaps more indirect, indications of possible links here might emerge from an appreciation of the associations between psychiatric state, social support and network characteristics.

The third hypothesis is that social support influences the course of specified psychiatric disorders once they are established. Breier and Strauss (1984), in their study of 20 patients discharged from hospital, found that 12 functions of social relationships were important in two phases of social need, convalescence and rebuilding. These studies have provided much information as to what kind of social support might be needed within the community if previously hospitalised psychiatric patients are to survive socially. However, they all tend to stress the fact that social networks of people with mental illness need to be strengthened or developed (Greenblatt et al. 1982) and in a variety of ways which might include ventilation, reality testing, material support, social approval and integration, and help with problem solving (Breier and Strauss, 1984).

Studies of many kinds emphasise a confiding relationship as being a key characteristic of the relationships within the social network in aiding mental health (Brown et al. 1975; Brown and Harris, 1978; Taylor et al. 1984; Eisemann and Perris, 1985). Furthermore, Freeman and Simmons (1963), Dinitz et al. (1967) and Lowenthal and Haven (1968) all emphasise kin or spouses as the key to an intimate or confiding relationship that is the most significant in terms of 'cushioning' the onset of psychiatric illness once a stressful life event prevails. However, the ex-long-stay hospital patients who are the subject of this study have such social histories or are of such an age that family members are unlikely to be so evident (see later chapters). If it proves to be the case that individuals' networks are devoid of confiding family members it will be of more than passing interest to ascertain to what extent such a vital function might be subsumed within ties with others within individuals' networks.

Carefully targeted intervention programmes appear to have the potential to help people to enlarge previously impoverished social networks. For example, in a study of a US hostel outreach program for homeless mentally ill people, Wayslenki et al. (1993) have reported that increases in social network size and improvements in network functions were related to clients being linked to other individuals and services. This was achieved through an assertive case management approach and illustrates the potential of linking formal and informal support systems. Brugha et al. (1993) on the other hand, in a study of a sample of people with long-term psychiatric disorders derived from the Camberwell register, draw a far less optimistic conclusion. Their results suggested that substantial improvements in patients' social networks could not be expected to follow either from improvements in individual social functioning or the expression of behavioural problems. Moreover, the findings did not suggest whether socio-environmental as opposed to personal factors were more or less likely to be the cause of severe deficits in people's social support networks.

Social network studies also tend to suggest that a more dense, homogenous network with strong, close ties (including family members) can provide more psychological support during a crisis period than a wide, dispersed network with weak ties (for example, Caplan, 1974; Walker et al. 1977). Baker et al. (1977) also found that patients who were released to family-dominated, emotionally supportive, secure networks had less severe symptoms of illness than those who returned to larger, more socially diverse networks. However, there is also ample evidence to suggest that long-term psychiatric patients tend to have weak ties rather then close ones (e.g. Pattison et al. 1979).

Furthermore, Baker et al. (1977) found that those returning to larger and more socially diverse networks in the community adjusted better socially and occupationally than others with smaller, more closed networks. Baker concluded that the optimal environment for returning patients would include both warm and accepting close relatives and confidants and ties to persons outside the family who could connect them to community life outside the home.

From an interim report of a longitudinal study of patients discharged from the regional psychiatric hospital (Crosby et al. 1990), many of which were in the study cohort of this research, it appears that long-term psychiatric patients under investigation: have few kin members with whom they have contact; have few 'friends' or 'confidants'; and interact with few people outside of the hospital environment. It might also be hypothesised that whilst ex-patients may develop ties with people living in the community who are unrelated to the psychiatric system, these may be weak.

Granovetter (1982) defines weak ties as 'acquaintances' who are less likely to be involved socially with one another. However, Granovetter argues that weak ties provide valuable functions such as the provision of information. In this connection Hammer (1981) has suggested that people with schizophrenia may in fact function best in the community with a set of distant social connections since these others can also offer feedback about behaviour in a manner that is not highly charged emotionally.

Persons with or without psychiatric symptomatology appear to have quite different social networks both in terms of quality and quantity. Greenblatt et al. (1982), Pattison et al. (1979), and Froland et al. (1979) all found that these were differentiating characteristics. Studies by Carstairs (1959), and Kreisman and Joy (1974) are among many which suggest that people with psychiatric disorders tend to be members of restricted and impoverished social networks.

Pattison et al. (1979) noted that persons who suffered no psychiatric illness were able to recall and list about 22-25 persons whom they felt were important to them and membership was diverse, including immediate family, extended kin, social and work associates as well as friends and neighbours. Psychiatrically distressed persons, on the other hand, had a decidedly less rewarding social world. They listed approximately 11 people, a very high proportion of whom were closely related to each other, over two-thirds of whom were relatives of the mentally ill person. These networks were therefore highly dense, thus restricting opportunities for weak ties to 'bridge' links to other social groups.

However, Silberfeld (1978) reported that mentally ill persons are less involved with relatives than are well individuals and that their closest relationships are with friends. This dichotomy is important as it indicates that although relatives may make up a large proportion of a psychiatric individual's social network, they may not be the most meaningful or provide the most functional links.

Although apparently restricted in some respects, the social networks of people with mental illness may prove to be important to individuals in other ways. This idea is supported by Dunn et al. (1990) who found that long-stay patients had meaningful networks which provided the patients with functions that were very significant to individuals within the context of the hospital environment. The 'strength' of these networks may give important indications as to how individuals adapt, via their networks, to particular circumstances and situations.

Nelson et al.'s (1992) interesting analysis of former psychiatric inpatients residing in different types of community housing found considerable evidence of reciprocity in transactions between residents and members of their social networks. Demonstrating reciprocity to be associated with well-being, the authors suggest that professional intervention which follows a paternalistic model can deny people opportunities for providing support to others. Like others (Carling, 1996), they argue that interventions which emphasise residents' strengths are necessary to emancipate people from dependency relations. It was also observed however that providing unsupportive transactions was related to mastery. Though apparently counter-intuitive, this may suggest that residents who are able to exert control and set limits regarding when and with whom they interact feel more in control of their lives. A cautionary note is sounded about the meaning of mastery in this connection as it is unclear as to whether this refers to autonomy, the ability to control family or other pressures, or other aspects of well-being (Nelson et al. 1992). Further research in this area is indicated. It was noted in the conclusion that the perceptions of residents' social network members were not sought so a truly transactional approach to understanding reciprocity was lacking. Further study of the functions and perceived meaning of reciprocity was highlighted.

Although writing principally about how psychiatric patients experience pathways through formal services, Spicker et al. (1995) report that in relation to social networks the 'most positive contacts were those in which respondents felt able to contribute something to others' (p.349). The reasons for this were not made clear although it seems likely from their later observations that this is tied to ideas about self-image and self-esteem. Regarding those persons with a fragmented sense of self, Spicker et al. suggest that 'discrete and uncoordinated services may confirm a weakened self-perception rather than restore a sense of personal integrity' (p.351). There seems likely to be a parallel with social networks here, meaning that networks which fail to make it possible for the individual to 'contribute something' to members of that network may in themselves serve to reinforce dependency and negative self-perceptions.

Uehara's (1995) review of Gouldner's (1960) classic statement on reciprocity is of relevance here. Uehara, adopting a deontological perspective, suggests that in seeking to explain the dynamics of social support it is necessary to look beyond social structural, economic, temporal, spatial and psychological factors, important thought these may be. She asserts that moral beliefs held by individuals enable, constrain and otherwise influence their interactions. Following Ekeh (1974) she criticises Gouldner for assuming that moral reciprocity obligations must be met by providing return *directly* to those who have provided benefit. She further provides evidence to show that the timing, focus and form of reciprocity can vary between individuals and that indirect and delayed reciprocity are common. More interestingly she concludes from the collective evidence in the literature that people tend to be more distressed by ties from which they 'overbenefit', i.e. receive proportionately more, than those in which they 'underbenefit', i.e. receive proportionately less. This has ramifications for research. For example, as Uehara herself suggests, it would be fruitful to ask questions about the range of moral norms or beliefs that inhibit people from accepting social support, or about what makes social support options 'morally available' to people even when physically and socially accessible. As yet, little research of this kind has been applied to people with long-term mental illnesses who may be assumed to face 'chronic indebtedness' in their social relations as well as social skill deficits or behavioural challenges in eliciting social support.

The emerging contribution of ethnographic studies to analysis of social networks and social support

Ethnography has been described as the most basic form of social research in that it captures the meaning of everyday human activities (Hammersley and Atkinson, 1983). Often called 'naturalism' (Blumer, 1969) ethnography has a long history (Wax, 1971) which dates back from the classical anthropologists such as Malinowski who stated that 'to perceive man or even traces of him and his works you have to be a trained ethnographer' (1935, p.3).

In a comprehensive overview of ethnographic studies, Hammersley and Atkinson (1983) argue that there is wide diversification in the definition and practical application of ethnography. Some writers propose the main purpose of ethnography to be the extraction of cultural themes (Spradley, 1980). On the other hand, researchers such as Becker et al. (1961) and Gumperz (1981) argue that ethnography's distinctive feature is the detailed investigation of social interaction. Still others suggest that the main role of ethnography as a research method is the holistic analysis of societies (Lutz, 1981; Fetterman, 1989), whilst Walker (1981) emphasises the 'story-telling' element of the approach. Finally, Glaser and Strauss (1967) maintain that ethnography is the principal way in which theory may be developed.

Ethnographers and anthropologists have tended to retain a primary interest in traditional bounded societies, but there are some notable and in this case very useful exceptions which have been concerned with modern pluralistic societies where boundaries are more fluid. Anthropologists such as Wallman (1979) have attempted to deal with this by making a distinction between what goes on within the boundary and what goes on outside of it. In a study of ethnicity and work Wallman uses the terms 'us' and 'them' to signify boundaries of difference. She argues that ethnicity as a process in which 'their' difference is used to enhance the sense of 'us' 'works' for particular purposes such as the mobilisation or enlargement of material resources and, particular to her study, employment (Wallman, 1979, p.3). Using Wallman's theory, one can argue that boundaries are at two levels. The first is the macro level in which ethnicity 'is couched in terms of culture, race, nation or religion'. The second is the micro level of 'individual perspective' in which 'the same difference may be described in terms of minutiae of behaviour'. At both levels, 'ethnicity is about the organisation of society and the organisation of experience'. This concept of boundaries is important to the present study because in the process of analysis, a central aim is to find out how it is that outside elements of the individual's existence e.g. residential setting, begin to mould certain elements of the structure and functioning of the individual's social network.

In the context of psychiatric resettlement it can be anticipated that potential boundary changes circumscribing people's lives have concomitant effects on what is experienced by individuals. Within institutions it may be argued, following Goffman (1961), that experiences or 'outcomes' for patients are largely a product of the service milieu for the reason that people are separated from family and informal supporters, employment agencies and community agencies. Within new community settings, however, ex-patients or the new consumers of services, are living in widely differing social milieux whose boundaries are probably much less clear cut.

Contemporary ethnographies concerned with mental health service users are relatively rare (Estroff, 1985; Barham and Hayward, 1991; Perring, 1992). Estroff (1985) has written about the experience of patients in the Stein and Test (1980) community model programme. Using methods of participant observation and questionnaires she described the experiences of a group of individuals trapped in a life which revolved around taking medication, stigmatisation by their own reference group, as well as by society at large. The study showed that the evidences of 'chronic patienthood' influence the amount and nature of social support. In particular, individuals labelled as 'crazy' lacked emotional intimacy and were confined to social support from mainly other 'crazies', volunteers and professionals whose support was limited owing to professional ethics. Furthermore, apart from paying taxes, most citizens have few incentives to interact with or help chronic patients. Barham and Hayward (1991) describe the trials of a small group of people with a schizophrenic illness living in the community largely from their own point of view, and in so doing attempt to throw some light on what social life means for them. Whilst most individuals were able to sustain contact with at least one relative who provided material and emotional support, they largely felt disconnected from a wider catchment of potential supportive relationships. This was tied up with notions of 'difference', some individuals feeling second-class citizens due to their perceived role as mental patient. Similarly, McCourt Perring (1993) uses ethnography to explore the experience of hospital closure from the point of view of residents. Her study found that individuals with long term psychiatric problems were able and willing, with adequate support, to make the transition to life outside hospital though the study focuses on the difficulties experienced by care workers in assessing and establishing the forms and levels of support which individuals need to achieve a satisfactory life in the community. What emerges from these studies, besides a graphic depiction of people's lives, is how factors can still arise which reduce the potential for individuals to lead fulfilling social lives.

Social functioning - an outcome measure of resettlement

Evaluative studies of community care outcomes have sought primarily to measure individuals' psychiatric state (Cheadle et al. 1978; Johnstone et al. 1984; Meltzer et al. 1994; Holloway and Faulkner, 1994). Such research has either found individuals' mental health to be characterised by levels of symptomatology (Johnstone et al. 1984), or to have improved (Jones et al. 1986; Knapp et al. 1990), or to have changed little since pre-discharge (Crosby and Barry, 1995). Links between these outcomes and the availability and quality of social relationships have been inferred (TAPS 1990; Meltzer et al. 1994).

However, the literature also makes reference to 'social functioning' as an important outcome measure of community psychiatric care (Hayes, 1989; Perkins et al. 1992; Reda, 1994). Whilst the term has not been comprehensively defined, it relates to rehabilitation in particular and also to social integration, both of which are discussed below.

According to Butler and Rosenthal (1985, p.38) rehabilitation describes an active process in which at least two people are involved; the person with a disability (the patient), and the helper (the therapist). They argue that to rehabilitate means: to re-establish, to reconstruct, to reinstate, to renew, and to regain. All of these terms indicate that rehabilitation is a building activity which attempts to: 'restore a person's physical and mental capacities and improve the quality of his life to a level which is, as near as possible, identical to that which existed prior to his illness' (Butler et al. 1985, p.38).

However, studies have shown that individuals with a psychiatric illness tend to be unemployed, single, rarely engage in recreational or work-orientated activities with others (Goldstron and Manderscheid, 1982) and have poor social and inter-personal skills (Wallace, 1984). There has also been considerable debate as to the causes of such deficits. Some writers have attributed the cause to understimulating and unstructured environments (Glynn and Mueser, 1986). Hayes (1989, p.57) argues that others have related disuse of skills to long-term psychiatric illness, cognitive disturbance, high levels of anxiety, or never having learnt them in childhood (Curran et al. 1982). On the other hand, Cohen and Anthony (1984) argue that measures of psychiatric symptoms do not correlate with the psychiatrically disabled person's skills (Halpern and Fuhrer, 1984, p.86). Similarly, Anthony et al. (1978), Ellsworth et al. (1968) and Englehardt and Rosen (1976) all argue that hospitalisation and drug treatment affect symptomatology, but have little impact on a person's vocational skills (Halpern and Fuhrer, 1984, p.87). Vitalo (1971) found that a group of psychiatrically disabled persons who successfully learnt interpersonal skills also increased in their level of symptomatology. Deficits in skills, including living skills (self-care, self-medication) and social skills (problem solving, meeting others, engaging in conversation) therefore are thought to relate to social functioning.

As a consequence, rehabilitation tends to be based upon a functional skills orientation aimed at optimising an individual's social functioning. Using the rehabilitative model social functioning therefore refers to the 'state' in which a person is able and has the opportunity to use re-acquired or acquired functional skills necessary to lead a lifestyle which is qualitatively similar to that enjoyed by others in society.

Within this 'state' individuals are also able to interact with others in a way that is meaningful to them and in which they may enjoy recreational and work orientated activities without feeling isolated or lonely. There is thus a clear overlap between social functioning and social integration, or the 'state' at which an individual is said to socially participate in the community.

Nevertheless, social networks may be regarded as the social conduits by which the above functioning skills may be transferred to individuals in the form of social support. For example, living skills such as cooking might be informally taught to residents as a part of household support. The social relationships through which care is provided and the way in which care is provided are therefore important for social functioning. Social functioning may therefore be regarded as both an outcome measure of social networks and social support as well as being a prerequisite for social integration.

However, identification of skills deficits is needed before functional skills training can be carried out. Within social care practice Lieberman (1982) states that assessment technology includes amongst others, interviews, self-report questionnaires, observations, and role-play situations. Anthony and Farkas (1982) argue that functional assessment instruments are categorised into measures of physical functioning, emotional-interpersonal functioning, intellectual functioning and global functioning as well as primary environmental focus (i.e. living, learning, or working). However, instruments tend to operationalise behaviours in the physical and intellectual area much better than in the emotional-interpersonal area of functioning (Anthony and Farkas, 1982). This was supported by the findings of assessments by care staff in the pilot study. Thus, as social functioning tends to take a back seat in assessments it may also form a smaller part of therapy.

This may explain in part why some evaluation studies of community care projects indicate that individual outcome measures of social functioning show little change from hospital to community settings (Perkins et al. 1992). Generally used instruments to evaluate social functioning include schedules such as the Social Behaviour Schedule (SBS) (Sturt and Wykes, 1986) (see for example Reda, 1994) and the Rehabilitation Evaluation Hall and Baker-REHAB scale (Baker and Hall, 1983) (see Crosby and Barry, 1995; Perkins et al. 1992).

Social integration and resettlement

The importance of social integration in relation to 'well being' has been advocated by many writers. For example, Durkheim in his study 'Suicide' (1952) suggested that rates of suicide vary inversely with the degree of integration. The idea here is that people who are well integrated into a group are cushioned to a significant extent from the impact of stressful events. Since they are regulated by the group, they are less likely to resort to extreme behaviour such as suicide.

Brown and Harris (1978) argued that social control and strong norms manifested in a high degree of integration could lead to depression and anxiety. Similarly Brown et al. (1966), measuring the overt manifestations of relatives' expressed emotion toward returning schizophrenic patients from hospital, found that amongst other factors, emotional over-involvement was associated with the return of the schizophrenic symptoms within nine months after hospital discharge. Thus there is a dispute over the relationship integration has with psychiatric well-being.

As previously mentioned, there is evidence which suggests that ex-psychiatric patients often wish to be with others of similar experience for care and support. The previous section has also indicated that relationships within a social network may also indirectly aid the development of social skills which mediate social functioning. It remains to be seen, however, whether, and if so why, individuals resettled from hospital to community seek to maintain long-established associations or friendships with their peers and staff, or whether the new opportunities created by alternative living arrangements lead to a restructuring of their social networks and the way they function to meet particular ends. These issues are taken up in subsequent chapters.

Summary

- Social networks may be regarded as opportunity frameworks of relationships which may or may not provide social support.
- Social support may or may not be beneficial to personal mental health and personal well-being.
- The relationships between social networks, social support, social functioning and social integration remain to be charted.
- How social support is construed by people with long-term mental illness is a pressing requirement for research.

2 Method - description and rationale

> The challenge for researchers and for practitioners of psychosocial rehabilitation is to develop methods and principles that reflect accurately the experiences, meanings and needs of people with severe persistent mental illnesses. The challenge is not to reduce the complexity of the task, but to make it understandable.
>
> (Estroff, 1995, p.87)

Introduction

In the introductory chapter it was argued that different theories about the cause and nature of mental illnesses can be linked to practical changes in treatment and care of sufferers. Thus, it may be stated that 'theory is a guide to practice' (Fetterman, 1989). Whilst 'a study cannot be conducted without an underlying theory or model' (ibid, p.15) so it may also be argued that there is a need for the conceptual underpinnings of the research design to be given. The aim of this chapter, therefore, is to provide the reader with a guide to the research process by describing the study method and rationale. A more extensive account is provided elsewhere (Forrester-Jones, 1995).

This abbreviated account will nevertheless illustrate some of the key methodological challenges that can arise, and how they can be dealt with, in the hope that this may be helpful to others entering this field of study. The structure of this chapter follows the guidelines set by Lofland and Lofland (1984) who state that although there is no standardised way of writing about research methods, certain chronological details are normally required. These are presented in the following sections.

Rationale - theory behind practice

It has already been stated that in order to gain a greater understanding of individuals' social networks a more holistic approach is desired. Since previous social network studies have tended to rely upon quantitative methods, qualitatively-oriented studies of the social lives and social networks of people with long-term mental health problems appear to be relatively rare.

Nevertheless, the holistic approach to research has been described as the most appropriate study method for an in-depth understanding of social phenomena (Mitchell, 1986; Denzin, 1970; Estroff, 1995). In order to gain this more holistic view of individuals' social lives, the chosen methods for this study were based on ethnography.

Ethnography which is 'influenced by anthropological theory' (McCourt Perring, 1993, p.2) has been defined as 'the art and science of describing a group or culture' (Fetterman, 1989, p.11). Positivistic methods are noted for their objective viewpoint of reality (Joseph, 1990). They are typically deductive in approach and 'establish a priori assumptions about relationships' (ibid, p.16). However, the ethnographer is concerned with describing and understanding the social scene from the emic or insider's perspective (Wallman, 1979; Khan, 1979). The subjective reality is regarded as 'no less real than the objectively defined and measured reality' (ibid, p.15). Fielding (1993) argues that as a method of first insight and discovery into a social process, ethnography is unparalleled.

This model of understanding reality is phenomenologically oriented. In other words, it accepts multiple realities. In this study, working from theories about the structure and function of social networks, ethnography was used to render accounts of people's lives, as far as possible from the perspectives of the individuals themselves. Participant observation, structured and unstructured observation were the main techniques involved.

This attempt to present a more holistic picture and gain detailed knowledge and insight into the experience of the people can often be lost in larger scale surveys (McCourt Perring, 1993). It was therefore hoped that the approach would help the researcher to move closer towards gaining greater empathy with the individuals and to understand them as people rather than 'subjects' or statistics. It was anticipated that the views and day-to-day experiences of the people themselves would become the key ingredient of the study, something which others have noted to be conspicuously lacking in studies of community mental health services (Huxley et al. 1990), as well as outcome and treatment efficacy research (Estroff, 1995).

The ethnographic approach used in this study incorporated many different types of research instruments. The use of different complementary methods is termed triangulation (Jick, 1979; Smith, 1975) and is basic in any ethnographic research (Fetterman, 1989). Methods triangulation in this study compared written, spoken and observed forms of data in order to strengthen confidence in reliability of the research findings.

Access to the field

Access to both housing projects was facilitated by new managers who welcomed 'outside examination' and 'feedback' of the organisational aspects of the projects. This may be seen as a reflection of growing pressure on professional staff to demonstrate accountability for their actions, and for health and welfare provision to be informed and shaped by relevant research findings (Hart and Bond, 1995). Such requirements within negotiations have been reported elsewhere (Buchanan et al. 1988). Dissemination of research findings allows clinicians and managers to make use of research avoiding the cost involved being wasted (Richardson et al 1990). In this study, feedback was provided informally at intervals during fieldwork. Completed chapters were then sent to each project and a presentation and workshop were also given once the study had been written up.

The relatively unproblematic access through the management level of the study housing projects highlights the advantages of researching new projects or ventures which are relatively unbounded compared to more established organisations (Bryman, 1989). Furthermore, related research by the Health Services Research Unit (HSRU) was already in process, the positive reception to which resulted in the privileged 'halo effect' (Fetterman, 1989) of being introduced to the residents and staff by the right people. This reduced some of the stress, fear, mistakes and insecurities reported to be frequent occurrences during early periods in a field setting (Stombler and Martin, 1994).

When we (the authors) visited each residence for the first time, we noted that each 'household' 'stage managed' the introductions in a different way. This illustrated the need to adapt initial field negotiations to the informal rules and norms in operation within each organisation. In this case, residential establishments which were driven by a common policy imperative already had their own distinctive ways of dealing with 'outsiders'. Different 'first encounters' with staff and residents also provided impressions of how the social milieu operated in different residences. This is explained more fully in Chapter 5 which provides an analysis of care practices.

However, in each case, it became clear that staff welcomed the opportunity for 'another helper', a role which was stressed as part of the participant observation element of the study. It was this that appeared to 'sell' the research to the staff, not only because it was less threatening than formal interviewing, but also because it seemed to indicate that the researcher was prepared to spend time and energy committed to developing an 'insider' view.

Access to information

The varied introductory sessions with residents and staff proved to be a foretaste of how dynamic negotiations at all stages and levels of research can be. Access to documentary information proved to be both easy and difficult depending upon the situation and persons involved. This also helped to shed light on how seemingly similar organisations operated in different ways.

Initial access to case files had been negotiated with the help of the HSRU during a pilot study at the hospital. Individuals' case notes were located in locked filing cabinets in the staff rooms of each ward. No problems were experienced asking staff to bring the researcher a number of files at a time to a partitioned area of the ward (used for patient-doctor consultations) to peruse and take notes on relevant information. Sometimes a patient would come into the area to sit and relax. On a few occasions, a member of staff came and asked the patient to leave so as not to disturb the researcher at work. There was an element of irony in this on two occasions as the patient told to leave was the person whose notes were being studied.

Case files were useful for gaining glimpses into the life histories of residents although information was sometimes missing, contradictory or both. Furthermore, documents written by doctors and nurses rarely reported situations from the patients' point of view, and so the validity of information was not always clear.

Although gaining access to case files at both community care projects was achievable, the response to the request was less favourable than had been received on the hospital wards. Case files for residents living in Greentrees were located in each house. Medical notes and life histories were normally locked away in filing cabinets in staff bedrooms whilst care plans and daily notes were usually kept on shelves or cupboards in downstairs dining rooms. Staff permission had to be sought to look at them. This differed from Mountain View where notes were all kept in an open filing cabinet in the staff kitchen. Access to these was through the manager. Strangely, within the projects, there was more reticence among staff and residents about the researcher looking through case notes than about interviewing them or reading the diary of the day's events. The following examples illustrate these points. The first was the response from the manager of Mountain View to a request to look at residents' case files:

Field notes 5 June 1991

R: Would it be possible to look at the residents' files?

M: Satisfy me will you - ask the residents themselves and if they say it's ok, then that will be fine... we operate on an open file system, but some of them are reluctant to do so... they find it hard because they are so used to them being closed.

This example is interesting in the sense that it gives an indication of the philosophy of Mountain View concerning case files. An 'open' file system was in operation which meant more liberty for residents to peruse their own case notes. On the other hand there was understandable reluctance about allowing an outsider (in this case the researcher) from having access. Efforts were being made to give residents a sense of ownership of their case notes so it follows that researchers should be expected to have to negotiate access to such information with both staff and residents. The seeking and gaining of approval from residents to look at their files did not in the end pose any problems. If anything, individuals were found to be apathetic towards the request.

Again, staff at Greentrees were uncomfortable about requests for case files. In many instances, staff would sit with the researcher whilst she was going through case files and 'talk' her through them. Others wanted to know why the information was needed and what was being written down. Similarly, residents would sometimes hover around when she was looking at case files, occasionally asking her what she was doing. This is exemplified in the following field notes:

Field notes 19 August 1991

> R:... George looked at me when I was reading the files. I explained to him what I was doing and why. He asked 'would it matter if I didn't want you to write things down?' I said that if he was worried about it then I wouldn't write anything down, to which he replied that he wasn't worried and that it would be ok for me to write things down.

This illustrates that residents had the confidence to express any anxieties they had about the use of personal information. It also demonstrates the need for sensitivity on the fieldworker's part to appreciate anxieties the researched may have. In this instance, with the passage of time, an open and trusting relationship developed, largely a result of an attempt to be honest, open, friendly and willing to join in both staff and resident activities. These characteristics follow the guidelines set by Neuman (1991, p.349) who states that '.... In time most people respond to genuine concern and interest in them', the goal of field research being to understand what activities and life events mean to those who engage in them (Baily, 1996).

Time management

Architectural features of the hospital ward provide a controlled and limited spatial arena for observation (Estroff, 1985). By contrast, the community has fewer geographical and physical boundaries and hence the reluctant resident could be difficult to locate. On one occasion, a resident with whom the researcher had arranged an interview had caught a bus to a nearby seaside resort. On another occasion, a resident the researcher had arranged to see had gone to visit a friend. Often when individuals did not appear at the pre-arranged time, the fieldworker would wait for a while and then go in search, often finding them in local cafés or public houses.

Lessons were quickly learned about adapting the research role to fit residents' less formally structured lives. In a world where routine had for the most part been removed, residents often created their own schedules. Although research projects are almost always time limited, timetables in which the researcher aims to achieve certain tasks in the day are not always within the researcher's control. Often, the unavailability of residents on any particular day resulted in 'early retirement' from the field. Sometimes no data was data. Timetables were still necessary so that goals could be met but the researcher learned not to get disheartened when these were not always reached.

Early on in the fieldwork, some residents adopted avoidance tactics or said that they were busy or too tired to talk. One resident refused to see the researcher, stating that she was 'sick' of answering questions from people who never helped her. It was thought best to respond to this by saying 'that's fine' and leave. A few days later, she apologised, said she had been feeling 'down', asked the researcher in for a coffee, and stated she would be happy to answer any questions that were asked. It is thus worth noting that whilst Baily (1996, p.75) recounts how rejections are common, and are not always polite, this need not be a total disaster. Rather, sensitive perseverance can lead to success.

Interviews

At the inception of the study, interviewing techniques were chosen which were suitable for charting social network data for individuals who had been long-stay patients. The Social Network Interview (SNI) was adapted from the Social Network Schedule (SNS) (Dunn et al. 1990) which had been developed and used in the TAPS studies. The adapted interview schedule allowed for a recording of the structural details of networks such as size, density, membership and interaction frequency. A more detailed description of the SNI is provided in Chapter 4.

It was found that although the SNI was useful for charting structural characteristics of individuals' social networks in a systematic way, it was difficult to tempt individuals into elaborating the significance of these social ties in their lives. A reason for this was that formal interviews reminded some individuals of the diagnostic or medical interviews to which they had become accustomed over many years. This is also claimed by McCourt Perring (1993) from her experience of researching former long-stay patients. Estroff (1995, p.83) describes how interviews, however unstructured and open-ended, fall short of capturing the real nature and significance of relationships for people with mental health problems. She illustrates how she accompanied one respondent to a church meeting whereupon she was able to gain a more fruitful recording of the person's social network than had been achieved at two previous interviews. Dworkin (1992) also discusses the special problems with interviewing persons with mental illness, such as their mental status, symptoms of their disorder and side effects of medication.

McCourt Perring (1993) asserts that formal interviews can reflect the mood of the individual on the particular occasion when they are interviewed and that 'a respondent may brush off a question or give inaccurate answers because she resents that particular question asked'. These situational problems of interviewing sometimes occurred when the SNI was being administered. For example, it was noticeable that the respondents became bored and restless after they had answered the initial time-budget questions. Qualitative data about social networks was therefore difficult to gain in this way.

There can be difficulties when respondents choose answers which they believe are socially desirable. Again this was exemplified during the SNI when the researcher attempted to ask the question about whether individuals regarded network members as their friends. It became apparent that after a while many residents tended to say 'Yes' to every question without pause. On the other hand, some residents disliked formal questioning about their 'friends' which they felt to be an intrusion of their privacy.

This highlights the point that formal structured interviews can arouse a degree of suspicion and anxiety. Lee and Renzetti (1990) argue that researchers require imagination, skill and tenacity if they are to successfully gather data in such a way as to reduce the anxieties of those being studied for whom the research may pose threats.

A further semi-structured open ended Resident Interview (RI) was later developed to identify network members not mentioned during the SNI and also to gather data pertaining to residents' perceptions of their own participation within their new homes as well as the community.

These short semi-structured interviews were easy to administer but in many cases the researcher resorted to memorising the questions and asking them informally over coffee.

Participant observation

Further data were gained by directed conversations with residents in natural settings like cafés and public houses, or in the communal lounge during the evenings. Since it was possible to stay overnight in the guest room at Mountain View, there were opportunities to observe and converse with residents at other times. Within these settings residents appeared more relaxed and concentration also appeared to increase.

Furthermore, visits to Greentrees were always accompanied with invitations to share meals with residents and staff. Involvement was extended in other ways. The researcher was able to accompany residents on walks and on visits to local cafés and public houses. She attended functions such as barbecues and went on outings to holiday resorts and major cities. This allowed her to observe dyadic as well as group interactions and helped residents and staff to get to know her.

The informality of such meetings posed some problems at the beginning because of the need to recall key questions. However, questions soon became familiar to her and, following the idea of Newby (1977), it was decided to carry a small note book around so that notes could be made in spare moments.

This strategy inevitably poses the question of whether the research was covert or overt. Although most ethnographers agree that qualitative research always meanders between the two (Burgess, 1984), the procedure adopted in this study was as a consideration for the respondents. Writing down information in front of individuals in cafés or public houses would have formalised an otherwise informal situation, and otherwise signalled another form of intrusion into people's lives.

After trust had been established it was possible to make use of a tape recorder during conversations. Transcription of recordings of these conversations and more structured interviews were invaluable for the construction of case studies. In effect it allowed individuals to join in writing their own case studies, a practice which Edwards and Talbot (1994) regard as significant to understanding experiences of participants within the caring professions.

Participant observation was also used to gain data from staff. Just 'being there' and joining in (though there has to be a balance between helping and seeing to be doing the job) was invaluable for gaining experience of what it must be like to live and work in the environment from the participant's point of view. This also enabled the recording of data from 'ad hoc' situations. The research process is therefore making the best possible use out of all kinds of data, including the use of unsolicited data which has been demonstrated to further understandings of social phenomena (Cormack, 1981).

Semi-structured staff interviews

The researcher purposefully waited to administer these interviews until the last possible moment of the fieldwork so that a high degree of trust had been built with staff. These were semi-structured open-ended interviews which sought to draw out details about staff perceptions of care practices. When and where possible 'creative interviewing' as posited by Douglas (1985) and Holstein and Gubrium (1995) was employed. This is where the researcher seeks to employ a climate of 'mutual disclosure' in which he/she is willing to share his/her 'own feelings and deepest thoughts' in order to 'assure respondents that they can, in turn, share their own "thoughts" and feelings' (Holstein and Gubrium, 1995, p.12). The results of these interviews are discussed in Chapter 5.

Scales and checklists

Rehabilitation Hall and Baker Scale (REHAB) and Krawiecka Rating Scale (KRS) scores generated by the Health Services Research Unit (HSRU) were made available to the authors and these are presented in Chapter 3 and incorporated into analysis in Chapter 4. REHAB is an attempt to measure the rehabilitation status of psychiatric patients whilst the KRS provides an objective rating assessment of the mental state of chronic psychotic populations.

The Hospital-Hostel Practices Profile (HHPP) (Wykes 1982) was used as the basis of gauging the rigidity of regimes of care in individual houses. Three of the original items in the HHPP were removed as they reflected features specific to rather traditional institutional practices which did not prevail at any of the community houses. The items concerned had to do with late night passes and special (hospital) shops. They were replaced with four items: being out alone in the community, pre-planned social activities outside the houses and domestic activities within them, and the requirement for set meal times (Appendix 1). Results are given in Chapter 5.

The Personal Presentation Checklist (Hampson et al. 1984) was used to chart the physical appearance of residents. It was anticipated that this would give some indications of the personal challenges residents might face when engaging the community. Results are described in Chapter 6. Finally, an adapted Social Integration Checklist (Shadish and Bootzin, 1984) was used to map social activities in which residents were engaged. The data were collected in several ways which presented opportunities for cross-referencing. Firstly, the time-budget within the SNI enabled resident activities during the previous week to be recorded. Secondly, since the checklist was easy to remember, the researcher was able to informally ask residents about their participation in activities. Participant observation over the fieldwork period allowed the researcher to develop a close awareness of the social activities of each individual. Findings are described in Chapter 9.

Analysis

Almost all of the qualitative data were transcribed and subjected to content analysis. Content analysis refers to the process of identifying, coding and categorising the primary patterns in the data (Patton, 1990). Both manifest and latent content analysis (Field and Morse, 1991) approaches were adopted.

Manifest analysis of transcripts results in a statistical account of the frequency of categories within the text. Socio-demographic and psychiatric characteristics as well as social network properties were tabulated and subjected to SPSS cross-tabulations. This method is often depicted as hard, rigorous and reliable since the data are precise and may be checked by another investigator. For this reason, it is often more persuasive than qualitative methodology and hence more likely to gain the support of policy makers (Bryman, 1988). However, others argue that such analysis results in data which is superficial and therefore weak in validity.

The latent analysis approach is one in which text is reviewed within the context of the passage in order to identify and code the major significant themes. Transcripts were read several times which helped strengthen emergent categories.

As technology advances, so research can make use of new techniques of data management and analysis. Social scientists have latterly begun to develop computer programmes to handle huge data sets with many variables that were once barely imaginable (Seidel and Clark, 1984). However, until very recently, these developments have been confined to quantitative data (ibid). Drass (1980), however, may be regarded as one of the pioneers in discovering the utility of computers within qualitative research. He developed a program called LISPQUAL which he used to reproduce some of the findings reported by Becker et al. (1961) in their classic qualitative study of education.

Gassaway and Elder (1981) argued that computers needed to be 'destigmatised' by qualitative researchers and 'sought to allay the misgivings that qualitative researchers had about computers, including the fear that computerisation meant a 'quantitative' distortion of qualitative methodology'. Following on from this, Seidel and Clark (1984) developed the Ethnograph in the course of their field work in a chronic pain control centre.

Using the latest version of The Ethnograph (version 3.0 1988) enabled efficient storage, cataloguing and analyses of data without using the more traditional manual cutting, pasting and indexing techniques regarded as the norm by many researchers (Spradley, 1979; Hammersley and Atkinson, 1983 and Lofland and Lofland, 1984). All taped interviews and informal discussions/conversations were transcribed into a macro within WordPerfect.

Once all data has been typed into the macro file it is then retrieved by the Ethnograph programme. Each line of data is numbered and can be coded and then sorted using emergent themes. A list of all sections coded with the same theme may then be retrieved and emerging areas of conceptual commonality and difference can be identified, representing a thematic approach to the analysis of data (Krippendorf, 1980).

The programme's obvious limitations lie in its inability to recognise human decision-making. There is also the risk of becoming mechanical about data coding and care must be taken not to stop reading or thinking about the text. However, the advantage of the Ethnograph lies within the systematic way in which themes may be coded, sorted and retrieved. This drawing of themes from qualitative data is synonymous with the grounded theory of Glaser and Strauss (1967) in which the importance of data developing theory is advocated.

For the critics of quantitative data, qualitative data is depicted as 'rich', the denotation generally indicative of the attention to intricate detail. Sustained contact with people also permits a penetrating or 'deep' account which can explore and illuminate the full extent of respondents' accounts of a variety of phenomena (Bryman, 1988, p.103). Whilst such analysis produces data which is of high validity, it has been argued that it may be less reliable due to the subjective nature of coding systems (Caldock, 1993). However, methods triangulation in which data from different sources are cross-referenced can help to increase reliability and validity. This is particularly true of case study analysis. Each case study of individuals or projects includes interview, observational and documentary data as well as researcher impressions, much of which can be cross-checked. Case studies were of particular significance to this research since analysis facilitated the search for patterns and themes within and across projects and between individuals. Therefore, a descriptive account of residents' social lives was provided as well as social network and social support properties.

Previous discussions of social research reflect a tendency to treat quantitative and qualitative method and analysis as two 'mutually antagonistic ideal types of the research process' (Bryman, 1988, p.93). Whilst researchers of one or other analytical type rarely deny the utility of the other, few appear to integrate the two.

However, it may be argued that the research problem should determine the suitability of a particular research method (Filstead, 1979; Scase and Goffee, 1982; Estroff, 1995). Whilst qualitative analysis is considered to be the most suitable for the research problem and therefore used extensively, quantitative analysis was utilised and where appropriate the fruits of both methods integrated. The result was similar to the 'structural ethnography' of Smith and Robbins (1982) who used an amalgam of quantitative and qualitative data in their study of parental involvement in Federal Educational Programs.

3 The community housing projects and their residents

> The influence of the settings in which people live may be very subtle...
>
> (Davey, 1994, p.194)

The purpose of this chapter is to set the research in its local policy and environmental context. Local policy for the resettlement and care of people with a mental illness is outlined. Two community housing projects are then described using documentary evidence. The philosophies underpinning both projects are profiled by drawing from interviews with management staff. Finally, outline details of the residents are provided.

Local policy for community care of people with mental illnesses

The County Plan for Mental Illness Services (1991) builds upon the health authority's earlier Adult Mental Health Strategy (1987). The influence of the 1989 Welsh Mental Illness Strategy and of the NHS and Community Care Act 1990 can be clearly seen in the philosophy guiding the County Plan and in the principles of service provision which it espouses.

Philosophy

The philosophy first of all asserts the value of the individual. By this it means that every person has a right to respect as a unique individual regardless of their status or contribution to society. This is interpreted to mean that individuals should have opportunities to live their own life in the community with dignity, self-determination and responsibilities. The requirement for an assessment of each person's needs, capacities and wishes is identified in this connection. The aim of services is therefore seen in terms of helping people 'to lead as normal a life as possible in the community', which is interpreted to mean, for example, 'the use of ordinary housing with visiting support in preference to care in institutions, and supporting existing social networks'.

However, the County Plan offers no clear statement about what kinds of responsibilities individuals would be expected to shoulder. Furthermore, self-determination and responsibilities may not be appropriate to individuals with very severe disabilities, at least not without provision of an infrastructure which offers mechanisms to empower individuals.

Perhaps the most clear policy statements are those pertaining to the use of ordinary housing. In the case of Greentrees, ordinary homes were interpreted to mean detached and semi-detached houses fitted with furniture and equipment comparable to what would be found in an ordinary household. However, whilst Mountain View was a large house renovated into flats offering modern facilities as well as privacy, due to its location and layout it was not unlike an hotel or office block (its previous use) and therefore its appearance was more ambiguous.

The County Plan also advocated that service users should be given opportunities to be involved in the design of services and in the formulation of their own care plans. It was recognised that a balance had to be struck between protecting people from avoidable harm and allowing them freedom and independence. The Plan stated its adherence to the principle of the 'least restrictive environment' as the basis for providing the necessary safeguards. However, whilst the theory of individual care plans sounds convincing, putting this into practice is difficult. Although the formulation of care plans was a requirement set out in the County Plan, little was said about the parameters involved.

Partnership with the community was seen as being promoted in a variety of ways by acknowledging that support for people with mental health problems is a responsibility for society as a whole, not just professionals. Services, therefore, had to be designed so as to offer support to and enlist help from families and other communities of interest who are connected to people with mental health problems. Public education was viewed as necessary to overcome ignorance and prejudice about mental illness, and close working was envisaged with volunteers, voluntary organisations and the independent sector in harnessing the reserves of the community. However, exactly how partnership with the community was to be operationalised was not spelt out in the policy documents. When the study housing projects are described in a little more detail it will become clear how, in the event of unclear policy guidelines, local projects can be left to make critical decisions about how best to mediate individuals' associations with the community.

A number of principles of service provision follow the aforementioned statement of philosophy.

Ways of supporting and helping individuals were seen as being based on the assessed needs of the individual rather than on traditional patterns of service delivery. Examples of the kinds of needs which might be anticipated included: help with problematic thoughts, feelings and behaviours; the chance to withdraw from everyday life; the containment of individuals for the protection of themselves and others; help with tasks of everyday living; social contact to create or maintain personal support systems; access to appropriate accommodation; access to generic and, as necessary, specialist resources dedicated to each person's educational, primary health care, occupational, and leisure needs; and access to advocacy. These are cited merely as examples but nevertheless give an indication of the components of what the County Plan refers to as a needs-led service.

In the interests of care which is coordinated and seamless the Plan indicated that each user with a long-term mental illness should have an appropriately skilled case manager, and that administrative boundaries should not present obstacles to the use of services. Accordingly, appropriate aftercare was to be available to all people when they left hospital or residential care, irrespective of their status as detained patients or otherwise.

Services were to be made accessible to all, despite the difficulties with poor transport, and it was acknowledged that there should be rapid service response times and efficient referral procedures. Linguistic and cultural factors relevant to sensitive delivery of services were seen as important. Accessibility was also seen as being improved by the development of up-to-date, comprehensible, locally available information about services and their aims.

The Plan reasserted a commitment to a service which guarantees the user confidentiality. Hence, users were to be assured that information about them would not be shared outside the mental health service without their permission, except where required by law. Information systems which connect information from individual care plans to local policy and operational planning were envisaged so as to ensure that the best possible and most up-to-date knowledge was being used. Staffing levels were to be sufficient to allow individual care plans to be implemented for each user. This involved making a commitment to staff development and to the support and supervision of volunteers. Services were accepted as having to be flexible to meet the changing needs of users and families taking account of changes in other services which are closely connected. Finally, the Plan underlined the need for monitoring and evaluation tied to an appreciation of service processes and outcomes. Importantly, it was accepted that there was a place for evaluation by users, service providers and outside agencies.

What emerges from this is the rather blurred nature of policy, leaving local managers with very considerable discretion in interpreting how to move things forward. Like national policy, it is relatively clear about the nature of global objectives but rather less specific about the means of achieving them. Attention is now turned to a description of the two housing projects, their philosophies and objectives. Some of the differences in policy interpretation between the two projects will become evident.

Two community housing projects - a description

Both projects were designed as resettlement schemes for people who have suffered from mental health problems. They were identified primarily for individuals discharged from Castleton Hospital and its nearby smaller sister hospital. Residents were able to stay at Mountain View and Greentrees houses for the 'rest of their lives' though it was hoped that a number of residents in Mountain View would eventually become capable of living in a totally independent environment. Mountain View was therefore viewed as an establishment from which residents might move on to even more independent living whilst Greentrees was seen as providing a more permanent home for individuals. This is a critical distinction to keep in mind.

In compliance with county plans, both projects were able to make use of the local community mental health team. This was a multi-agency/multi-disciplinary team established by the health authority and social services department in July 1990. The objective was to have specialist staff who would 'establish close working relationships with consumers, carers, statutory and voluntary agencies'. The team consisted of one rehabilitation officer, one senior social worker, a senior occupational therapist, community psychiatric nurse, project manager, deputy project manager, and team secretary.

Mountain View

Mountain View was initiated in 1987 by the Rehabilitation Team at Castleton Hospital as a response to the need for community housing for resettled patients. It can be seen as a joint venture between local authorities working in conjunction with housing authorities and voluntary organisations. A housing association provided the accommodation and the Health Authority provided top up finance. However, the local MIND group managed the day to day running of the project.

Physical environment

Mountain View was a large listed building with an adjacent cottage. The main house was converted into six flats; four in the main building, and two in separate 'cottages'. Altogether there were three single flats and three shared flats. Each flat had individual bedrooms, its own kitchen, bathroom and living room. The physical layout of the flats guaranteed that the aim of 'ensuring privacy and personal space' was fulfilled, this being written into the establishment's operational policy. There was also a communal lounge, staff kitchen, administration and guest room. There was a small garden to the front of the house and a larger walled garden to the rear. This rear garden had a lawn with garden seat, and vegetable plot. At the time of fieldwork, a greenhouse was also installed, as well as a shed for chickens. There was also a workshop adjoining the 'cottages' which was used for gentrification of old furniture.

Mountain View was registered as a residential care home by the County Council. The house itself was situated in the main high street in Castleton town. Two supermarkets were within walking distance. There were two bus stops close by. All public amenities including shops, post office, cafés, public houses and cinema were within walking distance of the house.

Staffing

Staff recruitment began in May 1990 and a manager and deputy manager were appointed in September the same year. Although both were previously employed by or had connections with Castleton Hospital, subsequent staff employed by November 1990 were appointed from many different backgrounds, including two former workers at the occupational therapy unit at Castleton, two former care assistants, one prison officer, a policewoman and a teacher. None of the latter were trained psychiatric nurses. This was part of the new philosophy in which workers were to be chosen for all the personal qualities and professional experiences they could bring to the job.

A staff development programme was made available to everyone. Only a few staff had formal qualifications connected to their work in the service sector. Therefore they were encouraged to take part in a day release course specially designed to meet the learning needs of workers in residential and day care services. The course was run from a university and led to a Certificate in Mental Health Care. The programme included modules on the use of self; the competent workplace; aspects of work management; teamwork; managing packages of care; working with groups; the role and function of mental health services; communication and assessing needs.

Staff consisted of eight project workers, of whom two were senior project workers, a deputy manager, manager, administrative assistant and a cleaner. At the start of the fieldwork, one employment trainee was working for 28 hours per week. This meant that there was a 1:1 staff-resident ratio. However, since a rota system was in operation, five staff were on duty during the day and often only one in the evening and at night.

Operational policy

The main aim of Mountain View was to enable residents to achieve maximum levels of independence (Annual Report 1991). From the inception it was hoped that residents would be helped towards independence, not only in terms of domestic living but also in managing their own lives. One way in which self-management was exercised was by encouraging residents to take some responsibility for making decisions about the choice of furnishings for their own flats and for the communal lounge. The same principle was applied to garden equipment.

Efforts were made to put in place a self-monitoring system by residents. This took the form of a residents' committee which met every month in the communal lounge. Residents were able to speak out about anything they were unhappy with or wished to change. An elected resident representative could also attend the Executive Committee. It was the hope that all residents would participate in the Residents' Committee although participation was optional.

Freedom of choice was encouraged in relation to the management of personal time. The right to say 'no' was also a feature of Mountain View's policy and was to be respected. In practice, saying 'no' meant literally that residents could refuse to participate in any activities if they so wished, including getting up in the morning. When fieldwork began, such behaviour was not necessarily viewed negatively by management as the following extract from an interview with the deputy manager attests:

> ... common practice in hospital is to get them all out of bed by 7 o'clock. Here, if you want to go and wake somebody up in the morning, you'll have to justify it. Why are you waking them up? If you haven't got any reason, you don't do it. It makes you think about them and not what's easier for you.

Independence was, therefore, tied to a way of thinking that meant individuals had a considerable amount of freedom to do as they pleased. Put another way, residents had personal responsibility for structuring their lives. This appeared to mean that much of the potential for leading more socially integrated lives in the community lay in their own hands. 'Anti-social' behaviour was looked upon as the individual's own charge.

Objectives concerning social relationships were also specified in Mountain View's operational policy. These included the encouragement of (i) the development of enjoyable relationships with others both within the project and in the wider community, (ii) use of general community facilities and (iii) involvement 'in the world at large'. It was hoped that residents and staff would develop and maintain close links with local community groups to facilitate the reintegration of residents into the wider community. However, there was no mention of how these objectives were to be achieved. Again it appeared that individuals were expected to take the initiative in these regards.

Five years on, some alterations were in evidence at Mountain View. Management had changed three times, those originally in charge having moved elsewhere. The present manager had been employed just under a year. Whilst staffing levels remained unchanged, five workers had been replaced. The Operational Policy document had not been modified but it was evident from discussions with management, staff and residents that the overall philosophy of Mountain View was different. Instead of the expectation that residents should take responsibility for their own day to day living as a sign of independence and an expression of their right to make choices, it was now regarded as appropriate for some residents to have help where they needed it. An example of this was with one particular resident who received help with cooking, cleaning and budgeting. Management reported that this had caused some consternation with other residents who were still perceiving Mountain View to be a residence where independence was supposed to be normative. Whilst daily structure had not been imposed upon residents, a 'loose routine' of social activities was arranged by staff. For example, tea was made for residents at particular times every morning and evening, and music, quizzes, hot pots and games evenings were planned once a month. The regime had become much more interventionist.

Greentrees

Greentrees Housing Project was a community-based residential care scheme designed for individuals who had been patients at Castleton's sister hospital. The project comprised five houses with three residents in each. Twenty-four hour on site support was available. There were five project workers allocated to each house, operating on a rota system. The scheme was managed by the local Health Authority, the housing was provided by a housing association and the project was managed by the local community mental health team. Each house was an unregistered residential care home.

Greentrees was designed as a 'supported living scheme' with an emphasis on assisting and supporting people to live in homes of their own. There was an emphasis on implementing 'individual action plans', comparable to those at Mountain View. These were to be reviewed every nine months. Greentrees also strove to prevent deterioration in the physical health of residents. Each person was encouraged to use an individual diary as a means of maintaining a daily log of what they had done. A house diary was made available to residents.

Physical environment

Four of the five houses were set within ordinary residential streets within the town centre of a picturesque market town. The fifth house was set in a residential estate about three miles away. Three houses were detached and two were semi-detached. Each house had either three or four bedrooms of which one was used for staff 'sleep-ins'. The houses also contained a kitchen, at least one bathroom, a through dining room or separate dining room and lounge. Each house also had front and rear gardens with either a greenhouse, shed or both. All five houses had also been furnished to a very high standard and had modern appliances such as televisions, videos and washing machines. Staff took responsibility for maintaining the houses, including interior decoration.

Staffing

Overall the project consisted of 25 community support workers, a project manager and one deputy project manager, the two managers being the only qualified psychiatric nurses directly employed within the scheme. Support workers were from different backgrounds and included a secretary, deputy headmistress, and residential care worker with children though most (15) had previously worked as either cooks or nursing assistants at Castleton. This was a deliberate measure agreed with the Health Authority in which the scheme would take on a healthy mixture of the staff from the hospital and from elsewhere. At least two staff remained on duty during the day, and one at night, within each house.

The principal criteria for staff recruitment were not so much nursing qualifications as 'life experiences'. The observations of the manager were instructive in this respect:

> We don't want particularly specialists. We've got the specialist support, haven't we, in the form of GPs, CMHT, opticians, chiropodists but what we want is generalist people who've got this life experience and again this common sense thing.... It was more important if someone was a member of the local sports team or was in a local theatre group. These general interests were very important. We weren't really looking for people with degrees and strings of A levels. That's what we had to think when we were recruiting - 'look tell us about your interests'. Just because you were a domestic or whatever doesn't really matter. If you happened to be chairman of the local golf club or member of the local council, it was possible to get a network there. That's the ideal, isn't it, that you use their network to tap into them, trying to get people like that who've already got networks in the local community.

Staff training appeared to be fairly minimal with project workers having a two week induction course, taking a compulsory first aid course and various two day sessions on fire prevention. No further training was envisaged despite the request of some staff to take the same Mental Health Certificate course attended by staff in Mountain View.

Operational policy

Greentrees's policy was based upon the philosophy of 'homeliness', with an emphasis upon the maintenance of individuals in the community. Policy objectives also included the implementation and review of individual action plans and the 'prevention of the deterioration of individual clients' physical and mental health'. According to the manager the main purpose of the scheme was to:

> ...enable 15 ex-hospital residents to live in homes of their own in the area ... very much this normalisation ordinary living... I feel we are talking more about life

> enhancement rather than out and out rehabilitation. It's not like they are 18 year olds or I don't see them cooking something by themselves or nipping down to Kwiks but they can play a more active role and have their lives enhanced more rather than, you know, do everything. I mean they are doing a lot for their age. You have to remember their age which doesn't go with a very active programme of rehab. Not that I think they should just sit back and get waited on because then the workers would just think of themselves as carers and that's no good.

Although the County Plan had stipulated the involvement of voluntary agencies, management had decided that this was something they did not wish to encourage as it contradicted 'normal living'. Similarly, it was felt that neighbourly charity was to be avoided.

Similar to that at Mountain View, the care ideology was based around enabling rather than direct care. However, in reality direct care was necessary because of the needs of some individuals. This is discussed in more detail in Chapter 5.

Five years on, Greentrees had expanded since its inception and included two more houses for younger residents. Out of the original cohort three residents had died. Staffing levels had remained the same but management had decided that there were surplus hours within some of the houses due to organised social activities attended by residents but not by staff. Staff were accordingly given other duties such as administrative work or sessional care work for other clients living in the community. Staff training had also been adopted. Care workers now had opportunities to take National Vocational Qualifications in Mental Health. Philosophy for Greentrees had not changed significantly but it was realised that with new and younger residents there would have to be more emphasis on rehabilitation to mediate independence.

Summary

In describing the two community residential projects a number of commonalities and differences have been illustrated in terms of philosophy and care practices. It has confirmed the literature which states that philosophy and care practice are not always symmetrical (Booth et al., 1990). It has also provided some insights into the way in which such asymmetry arises.

The description of the built environment and physical layout of the two projects showed that the County Plan aspirations for personal freedom and responsibility were adhered to in the sense that individuals could move freely within their own homes and experience a more 'normal' living environment as opposed to one of institutionalism (Pratt et al. 1980). Individuals also had the privacy of their own bedrooms to a certain extent. Although some individuals shared bedrooms at Greentrees where this was the case there was a separate dining room which could be used if individuals wished to be alone.

The overall impression of the projects from this description was that they were successful in gearing up towards community living. In particular, the Greentrees houses gave the appearance of being 'ordinary' in the sense that they were located in residential housing estates and of a type comparable outwardly to other local housing. This is in keeping with the general philosophy of integration in the community where small group homes are usually situated in residential neighbourhoods (Baker et al. 1977). Mountain View, on the other hand, had a more 'institutional' appearance. It was a large dwelling conspicuous by its presence in a busy high street in the middle of the town.

Whilst the philosophy and objectives of both projects follow the County Plan, implementation of the philosophy was sometimes a very different matter. In both cases, management found it difficult to strike a balance between philosophy and practice. On the one hand Mountain View's management sought to implement the philosophy without much deviation. This resulted in what could be described as a laissez-faire approach to the support of residents, with an emphasis on the rights of residents to self-determination. By contrast, the Greentrees philosophy of enabling residents to take personal responsibilities was rarely acted upon, apparently because of the advanced years and institutionalised behaviour of individuals. This led staff into direct care roles. The implications are reviewed in subsequent chapters.

Another issue to emerge from the foregoing descriptions was that there was much confusion over the language and philosophy in the County Plan and in operational policies. Comments from housing projects suggest that 'independence' has quite different interpretations and, consequently, a lack of uniform care practices may be expected. The nature and implications of such diversity for the social lives of residents are central concerns of subsequent chapters in the book.

There was also a dilemma with the training of staff. County policy indicated a need for trained staff. However, operational policy for both the housing projects was geared around staff having life experiences rather than formal qualifications. As we have seen, the projects proceeded to take up different positions on this matter, Mountain View management leaning towards adoption of a continuing education model for staff which was academically and professionally based, whilst Greentrees management disassociated itself from such an idea (although staff training has since been encouraged).

The emergent picture from the descriptions above is one of a local service which appears uneven (similar to that found by Renshaw et al. 1988) and dependent very much upon management interpretation of national policy. Two such contrasting projects in terms of philosophy and practice within the same locality mirror the PSSRU studies which suggest that care of the client group is characterised by fragmentation, reflecting the inevitable consequence of a system with agencies and professions espousing different goals and values (Huxley et al. 1990). On the other hand, the high staff levels in both projects were found to be an improvement on those reported by the PSSRU studies, (Cambridge and Knapp, 1988; Renshaw at al. 1988 and Knapp et al. 1992). Finally, issues of property ownership, patronage and compliance with house rules which sit uneasily with the philosophy of individual responsibility and freedom of choice also emerge as possible hindrances towards the policy goal of 'independence' but these are discussed later. Having introduced the housing projects, attention is now turned to the residents.

The residents

Information about residents in the two housing projects was gained from various sources. First, medical records at Castleton Hospital were used for name, ward location, age, date of admission and date of birth. These data were then cross-referenced with case files in each hospital ward. Discrepancies between the two were in evidence. Medical records tended to be out of date and lacking in essential details. With the approaching closure of Castleton Hospital patients were in the process of being moved as wards were closed down. A time lapse between the movement of patients and information sent to the medical records unit, coupled with the lack of information technology in the unit, contributed to the confusion. It was therefore necessary to visit each ward and ask the charge nurse or sister about the location of residents. Relevant information concerning individuals' historical and psychiatric backgrounds pre- and post-hospitalisation was extracted from case files. This proved to be a long and laborious job as case files tended either to be large and unorganised or in some cases incomplete.

The multi-disciplinary team assigned to assist community re-settlement also devised case files and individual action plans (IAPs) for each resident. These files were kept in the residents' community homes as well as in the team's office at the hospital. These became the third data source, again providing personal and psychiatric details including medication as well as rehabilitation needs and goals. Personal Data and History Forms (PDHF) of the Health Services Research Unit (Crosby and Barry, 1995) were used as a fourth source. Again, these catalogued historical, personal and psychiatric data. Finally, at the beginning of each social network interview, a further section on personal details was added. The acquisition of information from a number of sources helped to ensure cross-referencing in an attempt to minimise discrepancies in the final account.

The study sample of 25 individuals comprised 22 men and 3 women. This is similar to the gender distribution reported in Barham and Hayward's (1991) resettlement study where there were 39 men and 7 women. The present study group is representative of the wider sample used by the HSRU which involved 54 men and 8 women (Barry and Crosby, 1996).

Personal details

The average age of the sample was 61 years with a range of 37-79 years. Table 3.1 shows that individuals living at Mountain View were of the younger age group (average age 49 years) whilst those living at Greentrees were considerably older (average age 68 years).

The majority of the group (16 residents) were locally born (in the existing and neighbouring county) within Wales. The remaining individuals were born in different parts of England and Scotland. The study group was, therefore, variable in national and regional identity. Nine of the sample were Welsh speaking and stated that they preferred to communicate with staff in their first language.

Table 3.1
Age and Gender

	Mountain View	Greentrees	Total
Sample number	10	15	25
Gender:			
Male	8	14	22
Female	2	1	3
Mean age	49	68	61
Age range	37-65	58-79	37-79

Marital status is an important factor in the study of social networks and social relationships. Freeman and Simmons (1963) found that married ex-patients re-entering the community functioned significantly better socially and occupationally and remained longer in the community than their single counterparts. They reported that it was not merely the 'conjugal milieu' that accounted for the difference in performance but that married ex-patients had a higher expectation that they would perform well than the single patients. However, the majority of the sample (N=22) in the present study had never married and two were divorced. This in itself might suggest that individuals would encounter particular difficulties of adjustment when faced with living in the community.

At the time of the study none of the residents were in full-time employment but were in receipt of benefits i.e. income support and invalidity benefit. No-one had been in paid employment since hospitalisation. Prior to hospitalisation, twelve residents had worked as non-skilled manual labourers, five as semi-skilled labourers and one as a non-manual worker. Six individuals had never worked but three of these were in higher education at the time of their first hospitalisation. One individual described herself as a housewife at the time of her admission to hospital.

In British research, 'occupation is almost the sole criterion of social class which has been used' (Reid, 1989, p.6). Using the Standard Occupational Classification system (HMSO, 1991), two individuals were in social class I and II, seven were in IIInm and IIIm and fifteen in social classes IV and V. For the remaining individual, information pertaining to social class was missing from the data sources.

Since social class was defined using occupational status before hospitalisation it eliminates the possibility of monitoring the impact of downward social mobility on the course of psychiatric disorder. A study in Manhattan, New York, by Srole et al. (1962) used the occupations of parents to define social class of the respondent in order to rule out any possibility of results being affected by a decline in occupational level as a result of the psychiatric disorder. This was also done with the present sample. However, only nine individual files had recorded occupation for parents of residents. This sub-sample indicated that four of the individuals' parents were from social classes II, two from social class III and three from social class IV. Six residents had experienced downward occupational mobility, with just three staying the same. Such indicative findings question the use of simple self-report questions about social class which do not search out historical factors in people's work or family histories.

Hospitalisation

All of the residents under investigation had been long-stay patients, and had experienced cumulative hospitalisation for one year or more, with a range of 3 years to 46 years. For the group as a whole, the average duration of hospitalisation was 26 years. Eight individuals had also only been admitted to hospital once. This presents a cohort of people who have generally experienced continuous hospitalisation for much of their adult lives.

Table 3.2
Hospitalisation

	Mountain View	Greentrees	Total
Mean age first hospitalised	24 yrs	25 yrs	24 yrs
Range	18-38	12-42	12-42
Mean number of hospitalisations	9	3	6
Range	1-23	1-7	1-23
Average duration of hopitalisation	15 yrs	30 yrs	26 yrs
Range	3-35 yrs	19-46 yrs	3-46 yrs

However, more detailed investigation of the study group characteristics (Table 3.2) showed that the two community housing groups were different in terms of duration of hospitalisation and number of admissions.

Those resettled to Greentrees had been hospitalised for an average of 30 years whilst those relocated in Mountain View had spent on average 15 years in hospital.

Individuals living at Greentrees had on average experienced three admissions each whereas those at Mountain View had experienced nine, one person having had twenty-three admissions, exemplifying the 'revolving door' philosophy of multiple admissions which was particularly acute during the 1950s era of deinstitutionalisation (Jones, 1988).

Thus the individuals in this study who were admitted around 1940 and who had been in hospital continuously until their relocation to the community will have experienced many types of care practices and regimes and will have had different experiences of mental health treatment compared to those individuals admitted to hospital in the 1960s and 1970s.

The youngest age at admission for the study group was 12 years, the oldest 42 years, but the mean was 24 years. According to the DSM-III (1980) the age of onset for schizophrenia is usually during adolescence or early adulthood.

Diagnosis

Mental disorder labels have been shown to be significant in terms of how individuals identify themselves as people (Estroff, 1985) and how they make sense of their lives (Barham and Hayward, 1991). At some stage in their hospitalisation the majority (N=24) of residents had been diagnosed as schizophrenic (the other resident had been given the diagnostic label epileptic). The symptomology of schizophrenic disorders includes the presence of certain psychotic features during some phase of the illness. This involves symptoms of multiple psychological processes e.g. disturbances in content and form of thought as well as perception, affect, sense of self, volition, relationship to the external world and psychomotor behaviour, as well as deterioration from a previous level of functioning e.g. in areas such as work, social relations and self-care (DSM- III 1980, p.368). Individuals will tend to lack motivation, feel lethargic, and have difficulties in maintaining concentration on conversations, television or radio programmes or reading. Such symptoms should aid our understanding of individuals' desires to do little more than sit and stare into space (Howe, 1995). Onset of schizophrenia is normally before the age of 45, and duration of the illness will last for at least six months.

Medication

Medication is the primary form of treatment intervention within community based care (Barham and Hayward, 1991). Data referring to medications used by residents were collected from medical notes kept inside each individual's case file. The most commonly used drug was Procyclidine, an antiparkisonian agent. Twelve residents were taking this drug. This is none too surprising as most of the residents have been on neuroleptics or antipsychotic drugs for many years which can induce parkinsonism. Seventeen individuals were undergoing Depot Injection treatment. Apart from neuroleptics which are regarded as the main form of medication for schizophrenia, 27 other medications were also used by residents, including drugs for anxiety, insomnia and depression.

Twelve residents had also received ECT. Three residents had undergone a leucotomy. The study group therefore present as a group of individuals who have undergone many treatments for their illness and who are heavily reliant upon medication. Many also suffer from side-effects of prolonged medication and would complain about spasms and shakiness of their limbs. However, the most common side-effect which residents indicated was dry mouth. Only six residents were able to self-medicate whilst seventeen were dependent upon staff for at least the provision and regulation of medication.

Mental state

The Krawiecka Rating Scale (KRS) (Krawiecka et al. 1977) consists of eight 5-point scales (0 'absent' to 4 'severe') designed to provide an objective rating assessment of the mental state of chronic psychotic populations. Ratings are based on replies to questions regarding key symptoms during the past week as well as observations made at interview. The two scores are then summated. Questions relate to four psychotic symptoms labelled 'depressed', 'anxious', 'coherently expressed delusions' and 'hallucinations' (ibid, p.304) whilst ratings made by observation concern 'incoherence of speech', 'poverty of speech', 'mute', 'flattened incongruous affect' and 'psychomotor retardation' (ibid).

The HSRU carried out KRS ratings for their cohort in order for areas of 'disagreement and differences' in interpretation to be revealed (Mitchell et al. 1995). In general, the HSRU found that inter-rater agreement was satisfactory, in particular very high intra-class correlation coefficients (ICC) were reported for delusions (ICC of .81), poverty of speech (.78) and hallucinations (.99) (ibid). To gain scores for each individual in the present study, the total scores on both scoring sheets were divided by the number of factors (8 on each sheet per rater equals 16). An average score was then calculated. The results are presented in Table 3.3.

There were missing data for three individuals. One of these had died and one had been readmitted to hospital when the KRS was administered. The third individual was not part of the HSRU cohort.

It was found that seven residents exhibited very mild impairment with two individuals showing no depressive phenomena, whilst one individual showed a high level of impairment. The variations in numbers of residents in each category indicates a group of individuals with different overall ratings of mental state.

The KRS scores were then analysed in terms of symptomatology to identify in which areas of psychiatric state individuals were most impaired. The results are presented in Fig 3.1.

These show that residents of Mountain View were more depressed and experienced more delusions and hallucinations than residents in Greentrees who were more anxious, and had greater incoherence and poverty of speech, flattened affect and psychomotor retardation.

Table 3.3
Krawiecka Rating Scale (KRS)
scores by percentage

	Percentage	Mountain View	Greentrees	Number of residents
low level of impairment	0-5	3	4	7
-	6-10	1	2	3
-	11-15	1	2	3
-	16-20	0	0	0
-	21-25	0	2	2
-	26-30	1	3	4
-	31-35	0	2	2
high level	36-40	0	0	0
of impairment	41-45	1	0	1

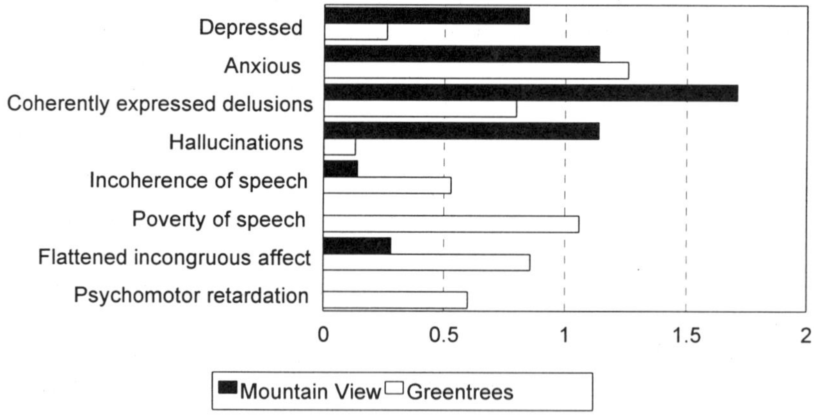

Figure 3.1 Krawiecka scores by individal factors
Mean scores low to high with high=poor behaviour

Observations and impressions of residents helped to validate the above findings. For example, Sarah of Mountain View told the fieldworker on numerous occasions that she 'felt down' in which case she would retire to her flat until she felt 'better'. She was often to be found expressing thoughts that appeared paranoid and delusional such as thinking that the hands on her clock were 'out to strangle her'. Similarly, Paul of Mountain View sometimes appeared to be hallucinating - staring into space and talking to someone not present. Investigation of individual KRS factor scores revealed that these two individuals displayed the highest hallucination scores (a rating of 4) compared to the rest of the study group. Ruth from Greentrees seemed to incorporate delusional ideas into her conversations with the researcher and was likewise found to have a high score (4) for this factor. Generally observations of Mountain View residents led the researcher to think that their symptoms were more acute (leg bouncing, fidgeting, heavy smoking, talking in the abstract, obsessional behaviour, pacing up and down) which may also have been influenced by the fact that they were more likely to state that they felt unwell than those at Greentrees. On the other hand, whilst residents at Greentrees tended to have speech skills deficits, they generally presented as being either 'burnt out' schizophrenics or never having been ill in the first place, not exhibiting anything other than signs of old age. These differences validate the KRS findings which demonstrated that the younger residents at Mountain View exhibited higher levels of symptoms such as delusions and hallucinations than the older residents at Greentrees. This was also substantiated by HSRU findings (Crosby and Barry, 1995).

Rehabilitation status

Studies of community care and mental illness conclude that rehabilitative success may be measured in terms of behaviour (Utena, 1978; Nguyen and Cebulski, 1987) as well as psychiatric state (Wykes et al. 1990) and that these variables can in turn predict levels of psychiatric care (ibid). Studies of individuals with schizophrenia have also shown that degree of social deterioration is only weakly related to persistence of positive symptoms such as hallucinations and delusions, the target behaviour of neuroleptic drugs (Caton, 1984). Dincin (1975) argues that rehabilitative models of care place a strong emphasis upon social functioning in the community and that individuals must establish normal social relationships if they are to integrate socially. Clearly, then, scores which indicate levels of behaviour are potentially very important to community integration.

REHAB or the Rehabilitation Hall and Baker Scale was developed in 1974 in the course of a major project investigating the effectiveness of operant conditioning techniques with chronic psychiatric patients (Hall et al. 1977). REHAB is used to 'assess the rehabilitation status of psychiatric patients' (Mitchell et al. 1990 p.40). It is a multipurpose instrument which identifies individuals who might potentially be discharged from hospital settings to less sheltered community settings. REHAB also identifies the most significant areas in the behaviour of patients so that rehabilitation programmes can be directed at the most appropriate targets. It can also be used to establish baselines and assess change in a patient's behaviour and disabilities over a period of time (Hall et al. 1977).

REHAB scores two areas of behaviour, Deviant, and General behaviour. Total General Behaviour Scores (TGBS) which are regarded by REHAB as the most important scores includes the following four factors: social activity, speech disturbance, self care, community skills. These categories are further broken down into behaviour types. For example, social activity is broken down into six items: mixing on ward, mixing off ward, spare time, level of activity, amount of speech, and initiation of speech. Hall et al. (1977) only regard the overall total General Behaviour Score to be relevant as it sums individual item scores and gives a balanced picture of the patient's behaviour. Individual TGB scores are not seen as significant when considering general levels of disability (Hall et al. 1977). However, in the present study it was relevant to look at individual factor scores to gain some idea of links between general behaviour and social network parameters.

The following table (3.4) shows the Total General Behaviour Scores for 23 individuals as well as the clinical judgment pertaining to the meaning of TGBS, six months post-hospital discharge. The scores below show that six months post-discharge, seven individuals were in the categories 0-10 and 11-20 which is normal or near normal according to the clinical judgment about the meaning of TGBS and a further four individuals were in the category 21-30 which is described as fairly good socially. However, five residents were categorised as in need of close supervision. Again, these scores indicate that the cohort includes individuals with very differing levels of capacity for independent living.

Table 3.4
Total General Behaviour Scores (TGBS)
with clinical judgment about their meaning

TGBS	Meaning	MV	G	No. of residents
0-10	Normal	3	2	5
11-20	Near normal	1	1	2
21-30	Fairly good socially Some areas need attention	1	3	4
31-40	Some potential for living out but needs training and experience first	3	2	5
41-50	Borderline potential for living out. Needs extensive training and experience first	1	1	2
51-60	Needs supervision to live out	0	3	3
61-70	Needs much tolerance and supervision	0	2	2

Greentrees residents exhibited poorer general behaviour with an average score of 38 than their Mountain View colleagues with an average score of 24 at six months post-hospital discharge. Corroborative findings were reported by the linked study in that older clients had higher overall dependency scores (i.e. total general behaviour scores) than younger residents living in the group home (Barry et al. 1992). The main conclusion to be drawn here is that Greentrees residents were on the whole more behaviourally impaired than their Mountain View contemporaries six months after hospital resettlement.

Closer investigation of REHAB scores was carried out in order to identify those areas of behaviour with which individuals experienced most difficulty. Results are presented in Figure 3.2.

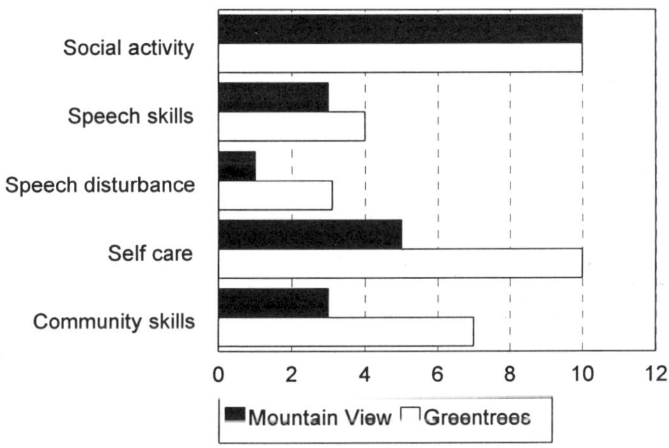

Figure 3.2 Total general behaviour - mean scores for individual factors Mean scores low to high with high=poor behaviour

The results indicate that although Mountain View residents had lower Total General Behaviour Scores than individuals living at Greentrees, social activity scores for both projects were identical. This is interesting in terms of the development of social contacts as it might be argued that social activity does not necessarily result in the development of relationships but that other behavioural factors are important for initiation and maintenance of network contacts. Furthermore, whilst social activity might be quantitatively similar for individuals in both projects, the nature and quality of social activity is important and raises the question as to whether social activity means merely 'being in' the community or participating in the community. These questions are considered in subsequent chapters.

Speech skills were less in evidence among Greentrees residents. However, there was a marked difference between the projects in terms of speech disturbance, self-care and community skills, residents at Greentrees displaying much poorer behaviour on these items. Again, these data can be interrogated in terms of the social network properties of individuals.

Summary

The group under investigation all had a history of long-term hospitalisation. However, individuals within the group varied in terms of age, mental state and rehabilitation status. Although the case vignettes (Chapter 6) give individual summaries of the social lives of individuals this chapter has illustrated some of the key defining characteristics of the group as well as differences in the personal characteristics of individuals between projects. The main points of contrast between residents from the two projects were that those in Mountain View were generally younger, had spent shorter periods of time in hospital and had better overall general behaviour scores than their Greentrees counterparts.

4 Social networks - an applied perspective

> ..... people neither truly experience nor act on the environment as separate individuals; instead, their experiences and actions are mediated by social networks.
>
> (Fischer, 1976, p.100, in d'Abbs, 1982, p.1)

Introduction

In the previous chapter outline biographical and clinical details of the study group were presented. Some indications were given as to the possible connections between personal and psychiatric characteristics and individuals' social lives, as previous studies have argued that the social and clinical functioning of people with schizophrenia appear to be linked to the structural and interpersonal characteristics of individuals' networks (Hammer, 1964; Cohen and Sokolovsky, 1978a; Wilkinson and O'Connor, 1982; Cresswell et al. 1992; Goering et al. 1992).

The social context within which people live is therefore significant to mental health and general well-being and is recognised by community care policy as constituting a key arena for assessment in its own right. In particular, opportunity for community contact is generally regarded as an important index of good quality care (Dilks and Shattock, 1996).

In this chapter, an attempt is made to assess whether or not individuals' social networks provide a sufficient opportunity framework for social support. This may be described as 'social embeddedness' (Barrera, 1986), or the actual connections people have to significant others in their environment (Streeter and Franklin, 1992, p.82). In other words, an investigation of 'social embeddedness' in this context aims to identify the direct and indirect linkages which tie individuals to others and which have the potential to provide support functions when needed. As outlined in Chapter 1, the opportunity framework may be partly or wholly functional, meaning that whilst some network members may provide support, others may not. The framework therefore refers to the formal structures (House et al. 1988) of social networks which include the parameters of size, density and membership.

Description of the structure of individuals' networks in this study, including size, membership, density and frequency of contact also provided an opportunity to investigate whether or not there is a relationship between network parameters and personal characteristics of residents. This also afforded an opportunity to re-examine whether the relative poverty of social networks of people with long-term mental illness (Pattison et al. 1975; Tolsdorf, 1976; Sokolovsky et al. 1978; Westermeyer and Pattison, 1981; Dunn et al. 1990; Cresswell et al. 1992) still holds.

The opportunity structure was mapped initially by charting the structural and interactional parameters of individuals' social networks using the Social Network Interview (SNI). The SNI follows previous studies which have used quantitative methods including structured interviews to elicit network details such as size and density (Pattison et al. 1975; Henderson et al. 1980; Brugha et al. 1982). The SNI used in this study was an adaptation of the Social Network Schedule (SNS) (Dunn et al. 1990). The SNS consisted of a name-eliciting procedure through a time budget inquiry of the previous day and weekend as a means of identifying any usual social contacts identifiable by name or role. It also provided an indication of the various settings in which contacts occurred. This procedure ultimately relied upon respondents' perceptions of their contacts. It stands in sharp contrast to that used by Dilks and Shattock (1996) who asked staff to record contacts made by residents on a daily basis for a period of one month.

Again, as with the SNS, the SNI interviews were also used to identify any other contacts in each setting and whether any letters or telephone calls were received. However, whereas the time limit of one month was used in the SNS, yearly was chosen as the criterion period for the SNI, reasons for which are discussed later. A family tree was drawn and residents asked to name and indicate where relatives should be placed on the branches of the tree. This proved to be the most successful part of the interview. Residents usually became much more interested and alert at this point, providing information clearly and succinctly, the visual aid presenting a break from questioning. The usefulness of visual tools within research have been noted (Beels, 1981) although have mostly tended to be used more as visual aids for the researcher (Fetterman, 1989).

Subsequent questions in the SNS (Dunn et al. 1990) were more concerned with the relative quality of social relationships in terms of a social hierarchy with confidant at the apex, followed by friendship, then acquaintance. This can be construed as a crude measure of social intimacy. However, this criterion of quality was limited in scope and orientation. Questioning was apparently geared towards the network members in terms of pre-determined labels (confidant, friend, acquaintance), rather than in the quality of possible supportive behaviours provided by network members.

The pilot study indicated that residents' answers tended to follow a response set, something that was not helped by the rather repetitive nature of some of the questioning. For this reason the data came to be regarded as questionable by the researcher. It was therefore decided that questions about the helping behaviours of network members would be added so as to minimise the tendency to respond in a set way whilst also moving some way forward towards understanding the functional qualities of different relationships. However, as discussed in Chapter 2, less-structured interviews and participant observation were the preferred methods to gain information about support behaviours so these were incorporated into the range of methods adopted.

Here, only the structural properties of individuals' social networks are dealt with, as well as one interactional parameter - frequency of contact. A more holistic picture of residents' social lives is provided in Chapters 7, 8 and 9 by drawing from both quantitative and qualitative data based on individuals' social networks.

The first stage in providing a description of residents' social networks was to quantify network structure. Size or the number of network members identified appears to be one of the most commonly assessed structural parameters of networks (Sokolovsky et al. 1978; Taylor et al. 1984; Cresswell et al. 1992; Goering et al. 1992; Dilks and Shattock, 1996). It is thought there is a relationship between the number of contacts and pathology with smaller networks being in evidence for individuals with schizophrenia (Cohen and Sokolovsky, 1978a; Pattison et al. 1975; Goering et al. 1992; Cresswell et al. 1992) than for 'healthy' samples. The structural property of size was achieved by simply counting the number of members named or identified at interview by membership category.

Yearly was chosen as the criterion period for contact because some network members, despite being seen only periodically, appeared to provide some important support functions for individuals. Few residents had contact with other individuals on a less than yearly basis. Those that were named but had no contact with the respondent were recorded but not summed. Hence a different criterion was adopted compared to that used by Dunn et al. (1990) and Dilks and Shattock (1996), both of these studies using a time budget of the previous month.

Network members were placed in one of the following categories: family, in-staff, out-staff, other residents, hospital peers, service contacts or social acquaintances. These categories merit some discussion. The category 'in-staff' referred to staff working in the houses where residents spent much of their day-to-day lives. 'Out-staff' was the label used to describe community-based staff working in local day centres as well as those within the local community multi-disciplinary team. Staff within the team included community psychiatric nurses (CPNs), social workers and psychiatrists.

'Other residents' referred to those whom individuals shared flats and houses with as well as co-residents in each project. Thus, for Greentrees, the category also included residents in the other houses. 'Hospital peers' referred to all contacts whom the individual knew from the hospital including patients still resident in the hospital wards as well as those now living in other community-based settings.

'Service contacts' were people in shops, post offices, hairdressers, and local community-based services who can be looked upon as representing community members standing in a formal role relationship to individuals. 'Social acquaintances', mostly neighbours, were those people who fitted into none of the aforementioned categories but who had some passing acquaintance with individuals.

Network structure - size, density, membership

Size

The number of contacts in each of these categories was then drawn out from the coded interviews using the search command in the Ethnograph. This acted as a validity check to manual counting. The results for individuals are shown in Figure 4.1 whilst findings for the size and membership of networks for individuals by housing project are shown in Table 4.1.

Table 4.1
Size and membership of individuals' social networks in two community housing projects

Membership categories	Mountain View Mean	Mountain View Range	Greentrees Mean	Greentrees Range
Family	2.8	0-6	1.2	0-4
In-staff	3.1	0-10	4.1	1-11
Out-staff	2.1	1-6	0.6	0-6
Other residents	5.7	1-9	4	1-12
Hospital peers	2.1	1-5	0.6	0-5
Service contacts	0.2	0-2	0.8	0-11
Social acquaintances	0.5	0-2	0.3	0-4
Total	16.5	11-28	11.6	2-46

These initial data show that, characteristically, individuals' social networks were small with a range of 2 and 46 and an arithmetic mean of 13.6 members. This is strikingly similar to findings reported by Thornicroft and Breakey (1991) who used the SNS to interview 80 long-term mentally ill patients living in inner-city Baltimore. They found that the range for the number of primary group members was between 2 and 48 with a mean of 13.1. Moreover, Dunn et al. (1990) found in their baseline study of 489 patients that the average network size was 8 members per patient. Similarly, for the 10 patients in their hospital observational study, the network size ranged from 2 to 19 with a mode of 8 and a median of 8. In a follow-up study of the same cohort published three years later there was found to be no change in the number of social contacts named but the composition of the networks had altered (Anderson et al. 1993). It was found that staff and patients named in hospital had been replaced by social acquaintances. This was explained as the result of a change in social contexts frequented by individuals who were now living in community settings.

In the present study, the mode or most frequently occurring number of network members for the group was six. However, as can be seen in Fig. 4.1, the size of network varies very considerably from individual to individual.

Network size varied appreciably between the two housing projects (Table 4.1). Those in Mountain View on average had larger networks (16.5), with six residents having networks consisting of not less than eight people whereas residents in Greentrees had networks as few as two and an average of twelve, with the exception of one resident with a network size of forty-six. This was to a degree predictable given that the two groups were of different ages, Greentrees and Mountain View accommodating residents with an average age of 68 years and 49 years respectively. As expected, many family members of residents in Greentrees were either deceased or were not in contact. This partly accounts for the network size differences between the two groups.

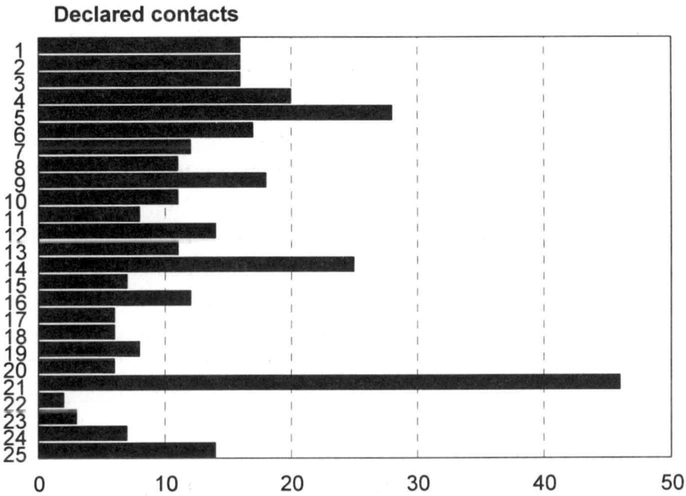

Figure 4.1 Social network size
(1-10=Mountain View and 11-25=Greentrees)

The two groups also consisted of individuals with different communication skills, residents in Greentrees being more disabled. Ragin et al. (1989) found that poverty of speech is a prominent feature of schizophrenia and increased after acute psychotic episodes. This would account for individuals in Greentrees having more disability in communication. They were, as previously reported, considerably older and had been under treatment for some form of mental disorder in hospital for double the time of their colleagues in Mountain View.

The psychiatric literature also suggests that people with schizophrenia have or are perceived by friends and relations to have pronounced deficits in social competence, leading to a loss of social contacts (Salokangas et al. 1991). Bellack et al. (1990, p.815) found that the individuals in their study were substantially impaired on verbal, non-verbal and overall ratings of social skills as well as on interview ratings of role functioning. Differences in communication capacity, seen in the context of the facility to initiate or participate in conversation, may therefore become a key factor explaining differences in network size for this study group. Moreover, poverty and incoherence of speech recorded for ten residents substantiated the point that some individuals had difficulties in communicating at interview. There is also the possibility that the communication difficulties of some individuals may have led to an underestimate of their social network membership. A discussion in Chapter 6 indicates the significance of participant observation in this respect, arguing that a more holistic picture of network size may be gained from a multi-method approach rather than a reliance on structured interviews.

Hospitalisation has been found to exacerbate social withdrawal (Wing and Brown, 1970; Lipton et al. 1981). It has also been suggested that there is a link between social withdrawal and the degree of social stimulation present in both the hospital and post-hospital environment (Vaughn and Leff, 1976).

At first sight, the data suggest that for this group social networks are limited in size compared to those of population samples which have even reported network sizes of over one hundred persons (for example, Sarason et al. 1983). Such a stark difference highlights even more that individuals with mental health problems can have very impoverished networks with regard to size. Although the opportunity framework for potential support appears at first sight to be poor for this study group, this needs to be addressed in relation to details of network membership.

On the other hand, some people may only need or want one or two 'key' supporters or confidants to sustain their sense of identity and well-being. In a comparison of the support network dynamics of 'three vulnerable groups': the old elderly, elderly people with dementia and adults with learning difficulties, Grant and Wenger (1993) contend that 'even within a large network the support hierarchy may be quite restricted in terms of its potential for substitutability' (ibid, p.95). Thus network size should not necessarily be regarded as a measure of network strength (Grant and Wenger, 1993). These points are examined more closely in relation to network density and membership.

Density

Density is closely related to size, and refers to the proportion of network members known to one another. Studies measuring density as a parameter of total social networks have been infrequent due to the logistical problems involved (Wenger,

1987). This is perhaps the reason why density has not featured as a measurement in large-scale epidemiological studies of social networks of people with mental ill health. However, the small sample used in this study meant that social network density could be analysed.

The importance of density as a means of understanding social networks has been well documented (Wellman, 1981). In this context, the density of residents' social networks would establish the extent to which individuals' social lives were tight-knit and insular. It is understood that high density networks are to be found in close-knit small-scale communities (Bott, 1957; Wenger, 1987) whilst low density networks are more representative of loose-knit large-scale (often urban) communities (Fischer, 1977).

In the present study the density for each resident's network was calculated using the network density formula of Brugha et al. (1987) but applied to the social network as a whole, not just the individual's primary group. Circles were drawn for each membership category from the interviews and names of network members were written into appropriate circles. The resident was then asked to indicate which contacts knew each other well. 'Knew well' referred to whether or not network members spoke to one another for longer than an initial greeting. A similar procedure was adopted informally with staff and other contacts. Since networks were small in size, this was not too difficult to achieve, and verified resident answers.

The formula used to calculate the density was $D = \frac{\Sigma N}{p(p-1)}$

D represents density, p the total numbers of members of the 'social network' and N the number of contacts known by each member of it summated across all members (Brugha et al. 1987, p.124). (Therefore, N is double the total number of links between network members as each is recorded twice e.g. A knows B and B knows A thus each pair is recorded once.) D ranges from 0 to 1.00 and can be thought of as the proportion of members within the social network that are inter-connected. The network densities of individuals are presented in Table 4.2.

The mean density for all 25 individuals was 0.7 but the mode was 1.00. This illustrates the fact that the sample generally had networks of very high density. A significant number (N=11) of individuals had very high density scores of 0.81-1.00. Fig 4.2 shows that 7 out of 25 individuals' networks had a density of 1.00, 6 of these residing in Greentrees. This difference between the two projects was somewhat expected insofar as structured activities within Greentrees tended to be based around other residents, hospital peers and staff which led in turn to a fairly circumscribed network of contacts.

Table 4.2
Network density

Network density	Number of residents
0.01-0.2	1
0.21-0.4	3
0.41-0.6	5
0.61-0.8	5
0.81-1.0	11

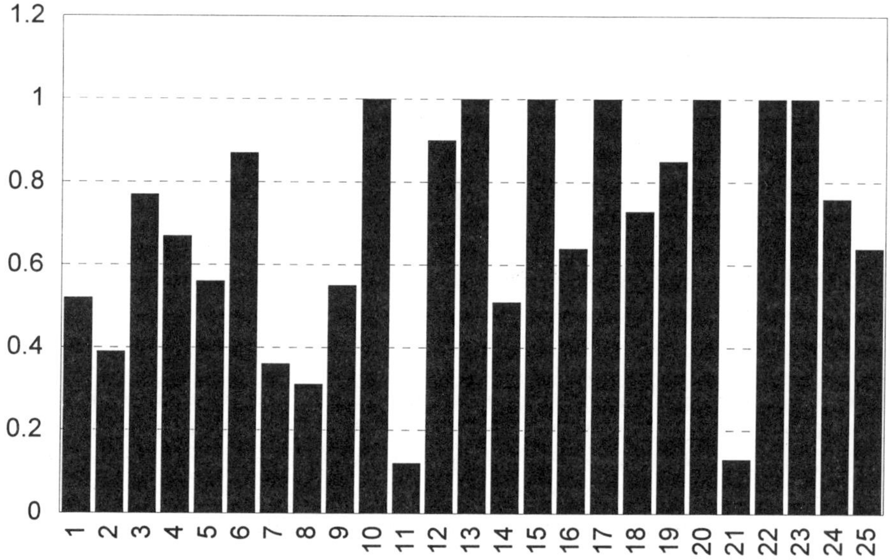

Figure 4.2 Density of each individual's social network

There was a very significant negative correlation of -0.6 (Pearson r) between density and total network size, confirming that the smaller the network the higher the density (Wenger, 1987). This may suggest that there is little scope for new experiences of relationships since most network members knew each other. On the other hand, high density networks have been linked to the provision of strong emotional support (Craven and Wellman, 1973). It has also been reported that members of close-knit high density networks are less likely to seek formal services in times of need (McKinley, 1973), suggesting that the network has an internal strength, or at least an insulating capacity. This is considered further in later chapters. However, the principal problem with network density scores is that high density tends to be biased by virtue of the methodology towards small networks.

Membership

The literature on informal support networks has shown a relationship between membership category and function within social networks. For example, the family has been regarded as the main provider of emotional and economic aid (Willmott and Young, 1962; Borchert, 1980; Anderson, 1971; Laslett, 1972; Harris, 1969) as well as informal care for aged relatives (Wenger, 1984) or handicapped children (Grant and McGrath, 1990; Grant, 1993).

Friends and neighbours have been reported to provide day care provision for children (Collins and Pancoast, 1976) as well as emotional and instrumental support in times of crisis. Service providers such as shopkeepers and barmen have also been reported as providers of companionship (Dumont, 1967). Likewise, fellow individuals who have suffered mental illness and hospitalisation have been found to provide each other with moral support (Sokolovsky et al. 1978; Barham and Hayward, 1991). Thus the membership category of support networks may provide an initial indication of the possible support functions available to an individual.

Residents' networks were characterised by very few family members (ten had no kin and only one had more than five family contacts as indicated in Fig. 4.3). Age and length of hospitalisation appear largely to account for this. Residents in Mountain View had slightly more family contacts (16 per cent of their total contacts) than those in Greentrees (10.2%) (Fig 4.4). There was significant negative correlation of $r=-0.43$ ($p<.05$) between age and number of family members, meaning that the older the resident the fewer the family members. Similarly, there was also a negative correlation of $r=-0.43$ ($p<.05$) between number of family members and years in hospital. Being an older group, residents at Greentrees had a much higher proportion of deceased relatives.

However, for both groups the type of contact by family consisted mainly of letter, eight residents receiving letters on only a yearly basis. Telephone calls from family members were received by six residents. Only ten out of fifteen residents reported being visited by family or relatives.

Hospital peers and staff were the most prominent members within individuals' networks. Individuals at Mountain View had more staff contacts than those at Greentrees (averages of 5.2 and 4.7 respectively). This difference was largely due to the care practices of the two residences, more about which is said in Chapter 5.

The average number of 'out-staff' members reported by residents in Mountain View (2.1) was higher than the average number of 'out-staff' per resident in Greentrees (0.6). This is interesting as the time-budget questioning found that 15 Greentrees residents attended the local craft centre and 7 residents frequented the day centres in Small Market. Hence, the potential for supportive relationships to develop with 'out-staff' in these settings was far greater than for individuals in Mountain View where only one resident attended Castleton day centre. However, participant observation revealed that the day centre and craft club had very low staff-resident ratios.

Conversations between staff and residents on an individual level were observed to be scarce and this might account for why 'out-staff' tended not to feature as members of individuals' networks. On the other hand, although residents in Mountain View did not in general attend local day centres, they did spend much of their time in local cafés. With Castleton being a small close-knit community there was always the possibility that residents would come into contact with staff known from hospital. This was also borne out by the observational work.

In both housing projects other residents and hospital peers were the groups most likely to be seen with an average of six members. Residents in Greentrees named on average four other residents. Whilst individuals lived with only two other residents, they did occasionally visit individuals in the other Greentrees houses. Residents in Mountain View named on average 5.7 other residents as network members. This was largely a function of day-time activity and daily routines which for the most part consisted of residents spending many hours in the communal lounge in each other's company.

On the other hand, an even higher level of network membership of other residents might have been expected given that they were living in such close proximity. However, conversations with individuals revealed that some individuals did not wish to be associated with their colleagues for a variety of reasons. This is illustrated in Chapters 7 and 8.

Finally, the strong positive statistical associations between the number of hospital peers and other residents $r=0.51$ ($p<.01$) as well as service contacts and hospital peers $r=0.41$ ($p<.05$) and service providers and other residents $r=0.50$ ($p<.05$) indicates something about the sociability of residents, as well as what seems to be the limited extent of substitutability and replacement of members between membership categories.

Mountain View was within walking distance of the local hospital which made it easy for some individuals to return to the wards and see 'old mates'. Two residents in the study still worked in the hospital gardens. This provided another opportunity to keep in contact with friends. Moreover, many individuals from the same hospital were discharged to various homes and hostels in and around Castleton. Therefore, there was a high possibility that they would have contact with each other in the town. In this connection, local cafés and pubs provided common meeting places.

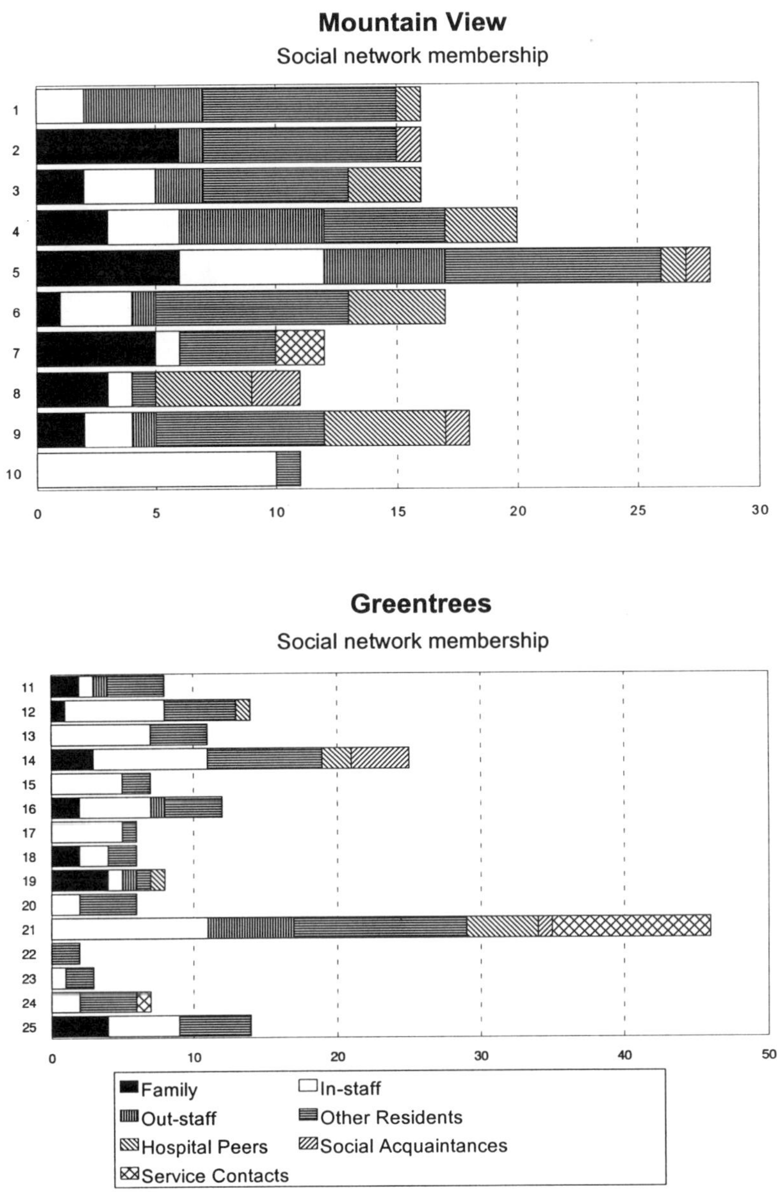

Figure 4.3 Network membership for individuals by housing project

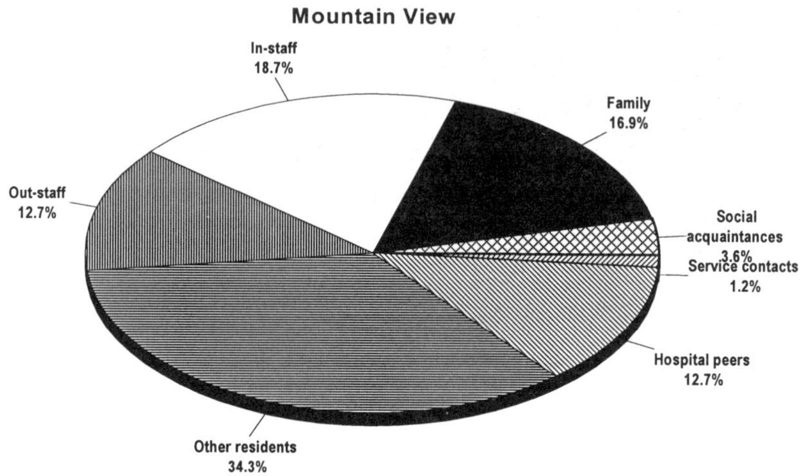

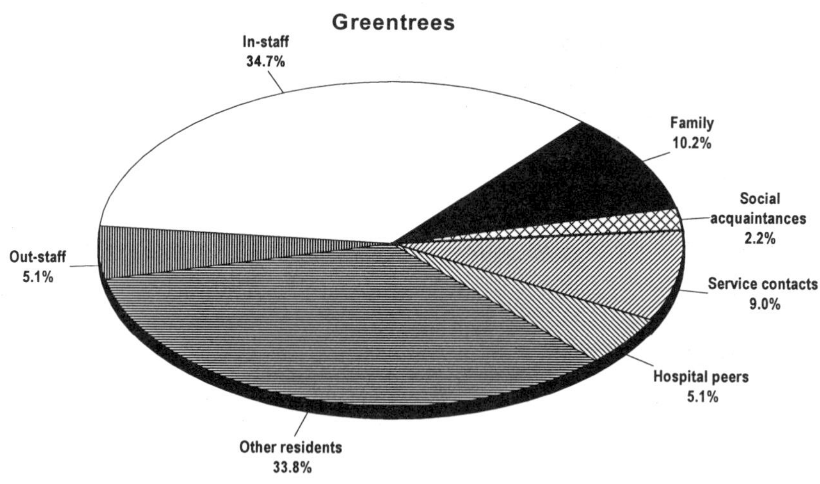

Figure 4.4 Distribution of network membership at two housing projects

Most residents (N=19) recorded that they had no 'service' contacts. Individuals in Greentrees reported more service contacts than those in Mountain View. This was surprising as shops and local amenities were much more accessible to Mountain View than to the Greentrees houses. Closer investigation showed that in Mountain View individuals' time was very much their own and was almost wholly totally unstructured. By contrast, time in Greentrees was seen to be more structured by staff around domestic chores. This meant that residents often accompanied staff when shopping, getting pensions, frequenting cafés and so forth. To some degree, therefore, service contacts were mediated by the nature of activities orchestrated by staff.

Different types of care practices therefore appear to be of key significance to the development of individuals' social networks. This is borne out in the psychiatric and other literature which demonstrate links between care practices and social functioning/performance of individuals (Barton, 1959; King et al., 1971; Bloor et al. 1988; Bean and Mounser, 1993). It has been reported that whilst over-stimulation of more independent living might result in negative social functioning and a higher relapse rate, as well as re-admission to hospital (Bean and Mounser, 1993), community care programmes aimed at 'maintenance can enhance individual performance, but do so through less intrusive means' (Huxley et al. 1990, p.138). The preferred option for care programmes would therefore appear to be ones which provide a balance between helping individuals to maximise their community contacts and placing them into over-stimulating environments.

Few 'social acquaintances' were named by individuals and 19 out of 25 had none. As already indicated, individuals in Greentrees on the whole did not frequent other places without staff. Although more 'service contacts' were seen to emerge, new relationships with other people were not in evidence. There was one exception to this. One individual named four people he had met in the church choir reflecting both the tenacity of the individual to return to an activity he enjoyed before admission to hospital and the encouragement of staff for him to pursue his interest.

To summarise, the data on network membership indicate that after six months in the community residents appeared to have made few new social contacts. Nineteen residents recorded no service contacts or social acquaintances. Individuals were still principally in contact with people connected to mental health services. Although there appears to have been little progress towards the social integration of people in local communities after they had been relocated, dislocation of friendships formed during hospitalisation appears to have been minimal. These findings are similar to those of Dufåker (1994) who in a study of long-term mentally ill individuals argues that the longer the respondents had been ill, the more likely their social networks were based on family relations, friends met through the mental health system and professionals rather than others (p.9).

Nevertheless, quality of life findings in the related work of the HSRU, which included most of the group in this study, indicated that 90 per cent of residents reported high levels of satisfaction in the life domain of social relations (Barry and Crosby, 1992). Barry and Crosby also found a very high proportion of residents who expressed high levels of satisfaction with their relationships with other residents (87%) and care staff (90%), with 47 per cent reporting that they regarded others in the house/home to be their friends. There was also a marked increase in satisfaction levels with the shift to community living both for relationships with other residents and for relationships with care staff. These findings suggest that whilst size and membership of people's social networks may be relatively impoverished, perceived satisfaction with the relationships involved may still be high.

Frequency of contact

Many previous studies of social networks have reported the frequency with which a respondent sees or is in contact with another individual (e.g. Irving, 1975; Toomey, 1971; Aldous and Straus, 1966; Horwitz, 1977).

Frequency was handled in the present study by noting residents' contacts with those in their social network on an interval basis. Frequency should not be construed as an index of the importance of contacts. It was possible for close and intimate relationships to be maintained over lengthy intervals when contact was not possible. Such persons involved, however, tended to be family members.

The bar chart in Fig 4.5 indicates that the most frequent contacts for individuals were other residents. This was to be expected as they all lived in close proximity to each other. Almost all residents, 22/25, stated that they saw at least one 'in-staff' member daily. The question must be asked why three individuals apparently had no contact with staff. The first person was described by staff as a 'loner' by nature and tended to stay in his flat. He often remained in bed unless there was something to get up for, such as his social security benefits on a Thursday. This questions the basis of the opportunity framework of some people's networks. If there are individuals available within particular, and in this case familiar, social contexts, does this mean that a network is poor if an individual shows little predisposition for social contact? On the other hand, the other two residents who did not recall daily contact with residents had problems with communication which may have accounted for their responses. The question as to whether network formation is a direct function of ego's personality or predisposition as well as the opportunity framework is an important issue and one which does not yet appear to have been roundly addressed in the literature. The case study analyses in Chapters 6 and 8 explore this theme further.

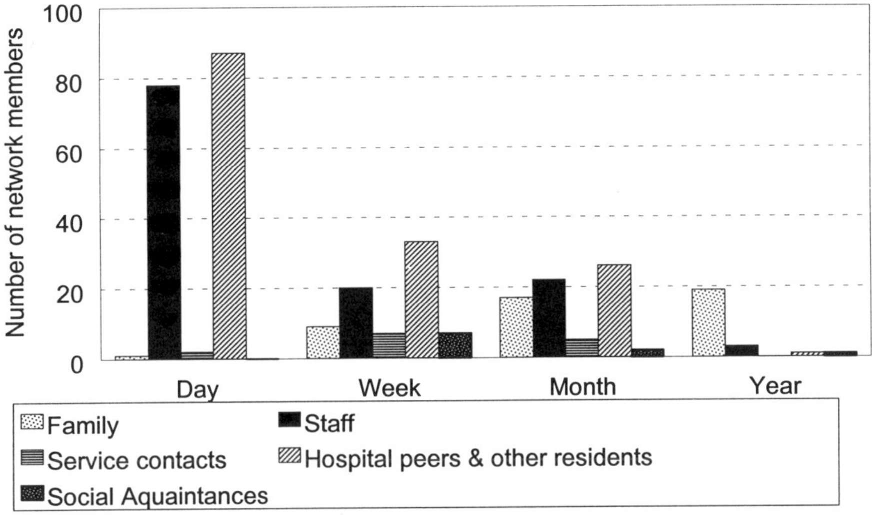

Figure 4.5 Network members in contact with residents on daily, weekly, monthly and yearly basis

Fifteen out of 25 residents were in contact with kin but only one resident was in contact with a family member on a daily basis (Fig.4.5). The average number of kin per individual was also only two. As expected, Mountain View residents had more contact with kin on a more regular basis than their counterparts in Greentrees. Frequency of contact with family members was on the whole irregular and based on long intervals. This is supported by the literature which states that family supports become eroded over time with severe chronic conditions (Eggert et al. 1977).

Only ten residents had contact with 'out-staff' i.e. CPNs, link workers, and social workers who formed part of the multi-disciplinary mental health team, and none of these were seen daily. They were mostly CPNs who came weekly or monthly to give injections, or social workers and staff at local day centres. This was a surprisingly low number as the operational policy for both projects stated that there were to be provisions for 'link workers' (who were part of the multi-disciplinary mental health team) who would mediate social integration. However, where there was an absence or limited contact with 'in-staff', there appeared to be some contact with 'out-staff'.

Staff and other residents were the people residents most commonly reported seeing on a daily basis. In terms of weekly contact, again residents reported seeing hospital peers and other residents but also some staff and a few family members. Only three residents reported having contact with social acquaintances on a regular weekly basis.

Discussion

In summary, most residents tended only to see other residents and 'in-staff' members respectively on a day-to-day basis. Contacts with other people, including families, were few and far between. People's social lives were as a result dominated by persons providing or using mental health services.

Interestingly there appears to have been comparatively little discussion of contact frequency in the psychiatric literature about support networks. The TAPS Project (Dunn et al. 1990) ascertained merely that out of a total of 489 patients the average number of contacts was 8 persons per patient who were seen at least monthly. Clearly the significance of these contacts, taking account of frequency, needs to be considered in the light of assumptions about the quality of relationships.

Finally, the data provide a limited opportunity to explore the connection between pathology and network parameters and to test further empirical evidence suggesting that residents can have an active social life despite the chronic nature of their illness (Sokolovsky et al. 1978; Dunn et al. 1990).

Inspection of Pearson correlation coefficients for the study sample showed an absence of significant relationships between social network size and KRS scores, suggesting that there is no necessary relationship between the severity of illness and the number of network members.

However, there was a significant negative correlation of $r=-0.4$ ($p<.05$) between network size and general behaviour (score from REHAB defined in Chapter 3) indicating that the worse the behaviour the fewer the network members. Furthermore, there was a significant negative correlation of $r=-0.4$ ($p<.05$) between general behaviour scores and social acquaintances. These data, which are indicative only, suggest that poor social behaviour may be related to difficulties in developing community relationships. Such connections are amplified in Chapter 7 from the perspective of the residents themselves.

Overall, social network membership for this group appeared to be much more restricted in scale than that for other population groups or elderly population samples (Wenger, 1984). There is indirect evidence to suggest that for older individuals this was probably the result of kinship losses through death or family moves. That is, it arose as a result of family life-cycle processes. However, in numerical terms, kin were shown not to be the dominant members of individuals' networks. This was a position occupied by other residents and staff respectively. Indeed, beyond these membership groups there was little evidence that other persons entered into individuals' social networks at all. This having been said, despite the restricted scale of individuals' social networks there was considerable variation in network size between individuals.

Although, at the time of fieldwork, residents had been living in their neighbourhoods for at least six months, few had developed any new relationships. Longitudinal study is necessary to establish whether community-embedded relationships emerge. For the time being it is nevertheless gratifying to record that relocation has not resulted in dislocation of people's social contacts. Although it was not possible to begin the network study before individuals were discharged from hospital, the social network data suggest that individuals comprising people's networks were much the same as they were when they were resident in hospital. This was partly the result of hospital discharge policy which sought to maintain friendship networks between individuals as they were moved from hospital. Put another way it could be said that community presence (O'Brien and Lyle, 1989) has been achieved but that community participation, as expressed in the form of new social relationships with community members, is yet to become manifest.

Finally, the adapted SNS facilitated exploration of data on a number of pertinent structural properties of people's social networks. However, this is only a start in charting the nature of people's social lives. The more qualitative aspects of relationships, and in particular the social support functions of ties, are more appropriately explored using qualitative research methods. This is the subject of later chapters.

Summary

- Findings for network size were broadly in line with those reported by other studies of people with long-term mental illness, that is they were much smaller than those found in population samples of other groups. Individual variation was apparent.
- People's networks displayed high density, a first indicator suggesting limitations to social contexts in which individuals could make new acquaintances.
- Network membership could be characterised as being dominated by other residents, hospital peers and staff. Family members were in the minority and community members constituted only a tiny proportion of the network. For the most part people's associates were those who provided or received mental health services.
- There was an initial indication that network size and number of social acquaintances were associated with assessed general behaviour rather than mental health status.
- Although attempts had been made not to cause significant disruption to people's networks during the resettlement process there were few signs that enduring relationships with community members were being forged. Subsequent chapters pursue this theme in more detail.

5 Care environments - their relationship to social network development

.... the survival of long-term mentally ill people in the community begins with the provision of structured and supportive residential facilities.

(Lamb, 1984, in Lewis and Trieman, 1995, p.257)

Introduction

In this chapter fuller accounts of the organisational structures and care practices of the two housing schemes are presented, building on the descriptions provided in Chapter 3. The aim is to show how these dimensions of community care can have some bearing upon the social lives of residents. Analysis of care practices and the underlining guiding philosophies and principles provides an opportunity to illustrate how staff perceive their role and tasks.

Mountain View - 'a step to independence'

The description in Chapter 3 presented Mountain View as a large house comprised of three single flats, three shared flats and a communal lounge. Organisationally the home was based around laissez-faire principles which appeared to reflect a commitment to 'responsibility for the individual'.

The principle of responsibility for the individual was operationalised through a system where residents had the freedom to make their own decisions and choices about their everyday lives. In practice this meant that residents could elect to do as little or as much as they wished each day. According to Carl, one of the staff members:

> ...of course a non-decision is a decision. They've spent all their lives in a psychiatric unit and decisions have been made for them... I help them to decide to do nothing on occasions and I help them to do things on other occasions.

Thus, care practices were characterised by minimum intervention to achieve specific ends. However, the limits to minimum intervention sometimes became much less clear, occasionally shading into a potentially neglectful approach. For example, waking residents up in the morning was regarded as imposing unnecessary structure. Hence, if residents wished to lie in bed all day that was accepted as their concern and right. Anything reminiscent of the rigidities and routines of the hospital environment was frowned upon with all eight project workers proudly stating that they had no daily routine. Carl once more:

> ...routine is used in institutions as a tool to actually repress people and stop their decision-making so I don't do that.

Even though 5/8 staff at Mountain View perceived themselves as rehabilitation workers, observations suggested that they appeared unsure as to what their role as project workers entailed. One person indicated that he did not really know what kind of care he administered and that he had never thought about it.

Others, such as Gwenda, argued that they saw their role more as helping residents to improve their social skills:

> We try to get people to do basic living skills for those who wish to move on or just to live here. We spend a lot of time talking, chatting, going over things, developing their interpersonal skills, trying to make the place look pleasant type of thing.

Others stated that minimal intervention was the desired aim. This is illustrated well by two other members of staff:

> You could on certain days do absolutely nothing from the time that you come in to the time that you go home.

> There is a lot of sitting about. According to the manager, if we are sitting about we are doing a good job. Everyone is happy.

These illustrations show that in the absence of any structured care programme, staff can take up different positions about the constituents of their role. For some it is something about which there has been little or no reflection. There were also uncertainties about the degree to which staff should intervene and the conditions which govern this. According to two staff members:

> I'm in a quandary. I should get Albert to do the cooking but he won't use the skill in the community and it is so much nicer and sweeter to do it for him.

> ...we can advise and suggest certain things to residents but we don't make anybody do anything here which is right but it leaves you banging your head sometimes because you are not sure what you are supposed to be doing you know. You sometimes go home thinking 'I've done sod all there today'.

Part of the philosophy of Mountain View was also geared towards what staff called 'individualism'. This was understood to mean that residents should as far as possible be autonomous rather than reliant upon fellow residents. In theory group activities were not encouraged. In practice, however, these were often the only activities organised by staff because they were considered to be more cost-effective than one-to-one interventions.

A key worker system formed the basis of any observable structure to care practices. Key workers were effectively the only staff that some residents such as Daniel, Jane and Sarah had contact with on a day-to-day basis. Their main role was to implement individual care plans, based on an assessment of residents' skills and their needs. Key workers were responsible for helping residents fulfil these needs. However, the care plan did not appear to be uniformly used, with 6/8 staff stating that it was not beneficial either because it was not fully utilised, residents having the option to spend their time as they pleased, or else it was deemed too ambitious.

Social integration was only seen as a prerequisite for residents who sought it. In such circumstances staff promoted integration by encouraging residents towards shopping, using public transport, and 'learning to relate to people'. They highlighted the opportunities for socialising by putting up posters about community activities and hoping that residents might go to events. Few did. There were different views about the practice of resident participation in the home. Six staff felt that it meant that residents could have access to all their files and were able to participate in the associated decision-making processes. There was a residents' meeting once a month which in principle was designed to encourage self-advocacy. This proved to be a successful way of encouraging residents to exercise their rights to decision-making within the establishment. However, practical participation in activities around the house as well as the wider social setting of Castleton was minimal. Two staff merely perceived participation in terms of involving residents in domestic chores.

The development of community integration was assumed largely to be the responsibility of the residents themselves as the following typical comment from another member of staff indicates:

> I don't see that we actually do anything to promote resident-community relationships. It's more what the client does to promote it .... Sarah might go to the pub for a drink on her own.... or the clients go shopping .... that sort of thing ...there have been a few problems with Gareth. We've got in touch with the

people and maybe explained what's gone on and have told them that if they feel that Gareth should be banned from here or there then they must do it because he is a normal person.

This quote illustrates the contradictions emerging from the care practices in Mountain View. Minimum intervention was legitimised by a commitment to respecting a person's individual decision-making responsibility. Facilitation rather than 'doing for' residents meant that individuals largely had to initiate their own social contact with others. Staff were guided by treating people as if they were 'well' individuals. 'Well' individuals did not need direct support and so this was rarely given. Staff perceived the residence to be a home for life for individuals but it was expected that some would move on to more independent living.

In summary, care practices in Mountain View were based upon notions of laissez-faire principles and the freedom of the individual to choose how to structure their lives. Staff exercised a minimum intervention policy but this left some members feeling trapped and confused about what this should entail and whether it was effective.

Commonalities of five households in Greentrees - 'a home for life'

In Chapter 3 Greentrees was described as comprising five houses, each one situated in residential estates in and around Small Market. Greentrees' policy was based around the philosophy of 'homeliness' within which the houses were to be regarded as residents' own homes. Residents were allowed their own possessions and had chosen and bought their own furniture. Bedrooms were decorated in different colour schemes and staff had encouraged residents to buy ornaments and pictures of their own choice to personalise the dwelling. This living situation contrasts sharply with life in the hospital wards where all furniture and sometimes clothes were communal and where, in a literal sense, individuals were never alone (Brinck, 1994). Care staff presented themselves as being committed to caring for residents as individuals and people with their own personalities as though they were part of their own family.

All the houses had diaries in which staff would comment on individuals' performance in various aspects of their lives from personal hygiene, domestic tasks, social and communication skills to activities attended. Each person had an Individual Action Plan (IAP) as a written record of their needs and goals to be achieved in terms of health gain or living skills. However, identification of needs took different forms. For example 38 per cent of staff said that they identified residents' needs by observation alone, 36 per cent said that they asked residents what they needed and 15 per cent said that residents told staff what they needed whilst 11 per cent said that they referred to existing care plans. Furthermore, none of the Greentrees staff said that the residents had devised their own IAPs. Eleven said it was the managers who had devised them, seven said the staff devised them and eight said that residents themselves had an input. With few residents participating in the preparation of their own plans, decision-making and control lay very much in the hands of staff.

There were monthly meetings which brought together staff from all five homes. Although informally organised, their purpose was for staff to discuss the physical, social and psychological needs of individuals and to report to managers some indication about progress being made. It was also a time for staff to ask and receive advice about any concerns they had regarding the residents or home management. There were also similar monthly meetings in each house which included managers, staff and residents. Informal discussions were geared towards residents who were encouraged to express any feelings or personal opinions they had regarding the home, the care practices or any activities in which they wished to engage.

In practice residents contributed little to these meetings apart from confirming statements made by staff about their own progress or problems. Staff did not attribute much significance to these meetings and stated that the limited verbal participation of residents was frustrating. It appeared that the staging of meetings was more symbolically significant to managers in making them feel that they were consciously thinking about the philosophical aims of 'ordinary living' than it was in empowering residents in any practical ways. Very few residents even mentioned the meetings. However, a strong commitment to philosophy resulted in the continuation of the gatherings.

Although residents were reminded that the houses 'belonged to them', they did not have the freedom to do as they wished in their own home as staff were ultimately responsible for the domestic running of the house. These conflicts may be regarded as arising from the adoption by the management of Greentrees of a 'family model'. This model is one in which the social structure of the house takes on the image of a 'family'. Variants of the 'family model' were in evidence however so a little more is said about these below.

'Hendy'

'Hendy' was situated in a quiet modern residential housing estate built on the outskirts of a small rural village approximately three miles from the town centre. There were no shops within walking distance of the estate and most of the other inhabitants were either retired or commuters. The bus service into town was infrequent and large stretches of the road were unpaved, making the route inappropriate for walking. Without access to a leased car, the household could be a very isolated place in which to live. At the time of fieldwork, Andrew, Thomas and Stephen had been living there for about one year.

Since the house was physically isolated from the town the household was fairly autonomous and took on a family structure representing that of the nuclear family. Each resident had their own set domestic chores which they dutifully performed each day. The house was regarded as 'belonging' to the residents and all of the staff stated that it was 'their [residents] home for life'. Homeliness was therefore emphasised through the participation of residents in domestic chores. The sharing of these chores was viewed as a route to developing a shared sense of place, responsibility and belonging.

All six staff in 'Hendy' perceived residents' acquisition of social skills as important for acceptance by the community. It was felt that residents could only begin to function socially if they possessed the social skills of manners and good eating habits. This was achieved by continuous instruction and prompting, usually at the dinner table which was the main focus for interaction between staff and residents. Staff also took residents out for a meal to a local restaurant at least once a week and on various day-trips and holidays. This fulfilled two goals. Firstly, learned social skills could be practised, and secondly there were opportunities to meet new people. At interview, half of the staff stated that they tried to increase residents' community relationships via personal presentation and social skills and half said that they did this by taking residents into the community.

The main symbolic boundary (Cohen, 1985) the household of 'Hendy' had to cross was acceptance from neighbours. Neighbours on both sides of the house ignored the residents and staff. Residents had also been turned away from one public house in the immediate area. One of the goals of staff was therefore to try and make friends with the locals as explained in the following quote from Morag, a full-time member of staff:

> ...it would be lovely if the neighbours acknowledge us and become friends. That's the big aim.

'Dayspring'

'Dayspring' was situated on a main road within walking distance of the town centre. Richard, Howard and Robert lived here.

Staff decided that the three residents should walk into town each day for exercise and to make contact with local shoppers and shop assistants. When residents went out they were encouraged to walk together rather than in a straight line so that they were less visible as being 'different' from 'ordinary' people. This social contact was deemed to be more important than domestic skills by staff and illustrated something about the philosophical underpinnings to their care practices. 'Dayspring' was characterised by a variation of the 'family model' in which staff regarded residents as older siblings. The three men were very much regarded as 'old gentlemen' by staff and their level of domestic skills was therefore not expected to be high.

However, since rehabilitation was an aim within the operational policy, staff tried to encourage residents to do small domestic chores like washing up and making cups of coffee.

It was felt by staff that the first step to community acceptance was personal presentation. Subsequently, the main form of domestic routine for staff revolved around encouragement of the three men to wash, wear clean clothes every day and take pride in their appearance such as brushing their hair. The second step to community acceptance according to staff was social skills. Instruction by staff again was concentrated around meal times.

Staff felt under pressure to present the three residents in a manner that was acceptable to the community as shown in the following statement by Norma:

> I feel there is a pressure to compensate for who they are. At home I get up in the morning. If I've done the washing the night before and I want to put my dressing gown and slippers on and go and hang my washing out I will do it. Now if one of these (residents) went in the garden in a dressing gown and slippers... it just wouldn't be accepted. It's double standards. Nobody would bat an eye if I did it.

In terms of community social integration, staff regarded the three men to have been accepted by the neighbours. This was particularly true of one neighbour who had originally set up a petition against 'ex-patients' moving into the neighbourhood, but who was subsequently friendly to the three men as a result of Richard mowing her lawn.

The family model of care was also apparent from observations of 'Dayspring'. Staff regarded the three men as childlike. This is exemplified in the following quote from another member of staff, Jessica:

> We regard our roles as carers like home helps, nurturing roles... Richard is sometimes like a five year old... you chastise, you encourage, you're boosting and building their self-confidence... if we are going out for a day we tend to say we'll have a family outing. We tend to use words like that. We refer to each other not as another member of staff but by Christian names.

This comment illustrates that staff used the family model to structure their activities and to make sense of those they were caring for.

'Woodlands'

'Woodlands' was situated along a main road leading out of Small Market. Timothy, Walter and Sidney lived here. There were no specific routines in this house, 4/5 staff said that they had no routine nor wanted one. The main guiding principle adopted by staff was 'freedom of choice' and 'residents' rights. There was a strong feeling that residents ought to be allowed to exercise the veto in regard to participation in activities. 'Keeping them company' was felt to be very important and the main role of project workers. Hence, staff socialised with the residents by watching television with the three men, playing games, and going on outings. It was felt by staff that since residents were living in the community, they were part of the community. The main idea was that they should be happy with what they were doing. Social skills and personal presentation were therefore not deemed to be of prime importance.

In this house staff viewed their role as younger relatives caring for their older kin rather than a maternal role discernible in 'Hendy' or a sibling role found in 'Dayspring'. This was exemplified in a quote by Gwil:

> ... the care we give is what they would expect from their own family really if they were there to care for them. I think that's important. Trying to give the care their relatives would have given had they maybe been alive...

Whilst staff did most of the domestic work in the house the three men liked to wash up together. Sidney would clear the table, Timothy would scrape the dirty plates, wash pots and pans and Walter would dry the dishes. This 'human conveyor belt' consisting of the three men silently and slowly going about their tasks and taking pride in doing it properly was fascinating to observe and illustrated how performing even the simplest of tasks could evoke a sense of worth. Walter asked the staff to tell him when it was time to do this and became upset if he was left out. It therefore appeared that these roles were a vitally important part of these men's lives. Timothy had also taken charge of the garden and grew tomatoes and lettuce in his greenhouse.

Community integration was not a major priority for the staff in 'Woodlands'. They felt that it was important that people talked to the three men but that they should not be 'forced into relationships'. Like 'Hendy' the residents in 'Woodlands' were not welcomed by the neighbours when they first moved in but with the passage of time they appeared to have become more accepted.

The household at 'Woodlands' was therefore characterised by a model in which staff regarded residents as older relatives. There was very little contact with others outside of the house.

'Cliffton'

'Cliffton' was semi-detached and situated on a busy main road approximately half a mile out of Small Market. James, Ruth and Owain lived here.

There appeared not to be any one principle guiding the organisational structure of 'Cliffton'. Rather there were two to some extent counterposing principles which could be regarded respectively as interventionist and laissez-faire.

The principle of laissez-faire was mirrored in the fact that the only visible evidence of routine was set meal times. Ruth and Owain tended to spend large amounts of time in the lounge watching the television. James, the more active of the three, had made his own routine geared around activities such as the day centre and art club.

The interventionist policy was evident by the fact that staff carried out almost all domestic activities (4/5 stating that they viewed their role as housekeeper) with little resident participation. This may be regarded as dependency inducing though staff felt that their 'clients' had needs for which intervention was necessary. These included bathing, clothing and cooking. Residents each had their own things to do in the house. James would lay the table, take out the bins and pay the milkman. Ruth would help to clear away the dishes and Owain had recently learned how to make a cup of tea. Staff were frustrated at the slow progress their residents had made in terms of domestic participation. However they also stated that Ruth was very frail and Owain engaged in very little verbal communication. Staff felt that any form of rehabilitation would therefore be a gradual process and that the residents should not be pushed. However, since the three residents were 'mixed-ability' in terms of social functioning, this appeared to result in Owain receiving less attention than the other two because he rarely communicated and spoke in monosyllables. Rehabilitation was based around social skills training including manners and personal hygiene.

Since staff and residents spent a lot of time in the house they got to know the neighbours next door very well. They watched the house for their neighbours when they went away and received post-cards from them. Staff felt that this showed an important degree of mutual trust.

Staff would have liked more people from the community to visit the residents. As one member of staff commented in this regard:

> It would be really nice if there was someone from the end of this street who would call to see them for a cup of tea or take them out somewhere. Just to be an ordinary member of the community, not people seeing them as someone different.

Life at 'Cliffton' was rather self-contained though still based upon a variant of the family model. There was a strong laissez-faire element underpinning some practices, coupled with a tendency to interventionism where staff 'took over' domestic activities.

'Brangwyn'

'Brangwyn' was detached and situated in a modern residential estate within a short walking distance from the town centre. The household was regarded by staff to be 'high dependency', the residents, Matthew, Edward and Frederick, who lived there having specific needs. Frederick was partially sighted, Matthew had problems with personal mobility and Edward had social problems with children in town who taunted him. Matthew and Frederick also presented as a safety risk, the two having previously set themselves alight with cigarettes and a pipe.

Routines were based primarily around the physical care of two individuals and also domestic chores. Prompting was used to try and improve residents' social skills and, although there was very little participation by residents, each had a role to play which was made significant for them by constant praise from staff.

Verbal interaction between staff and residents was more in evidence at 'Brangwyn' than in any of the other houses. The atmosphere was very light-hearted and there was much laughter and joking. The main principle generally guiding this house was interventionist with staff engaged most of the time in domestic and physical care. Staff regarded residents as needing 'child care' and very close staff-resident relationships were formed.

Models of care

Geertz (1973) argues that models are 'maps for' rather than 'maps of' social phenomena. Social scientists use models to build up a theoretical picture of what is happening within a social situation (McCourt Perring 1993). In this study, models of care are used to understand how and why organisations (in this instance community housing projects) structure and deliver support or care to individuals. They may also provide pointers about how different care practices mediate the development of social networks.

From the profiles of Greentrees presented above, variants of the family model were discerned. These included the 'homely' model ('Hendy') in which a sense of 'belonging' guided care practices and social activities; the quasi-sibling model ('Dayspring') in which staff saw their role as older brothers and sisters and the kinship model ('Woodlands') in which staff regarded residents as older relatives. The fourth type of model discernible from the data was one based on interventionist principles ('Brangwyn') in which staff took on more of a maternal nursing care role (this was something akin to the medical model). The fifth variant ('Cliffton') was one in which intervention varied in its relative emphasis on domesticity, physical care and social activities. Mountain View operated within the model of care based upon laissez-faire principles though was further along the continuum of 'complete freedom of choice' for the individual than was 'Cliffton'.

Having briefly outlined the different models of care, attention is now turned to factors associated with these models.

Perceived roles

The question, 'how do you see your position as carer?' generated five different responses which included the practicalities of care or 'tending', including care/nursing, domestic/housekeeper and rehabilitation worker, as well as emotional supportive roles such as friend and quasi-relative. Staff tended to perceive themselves as part of a family structure. Twelve of the 26 Greentrees staff described themselves as 'housekeepers' or 'domestics', whilst two also stated that they viewed their position as a rehabilitation worker, and five 'as if' nurses. However, eight stated that they saw their primary roles as friends of the residents, and two regarded themselves as quasi-relatives. Therefore, although a high percentage of staff (38%) believed themselves to occupy informal type roles (friends and relatives), in general they saw their role as that of a paid housekeeper.

Staff in 'Brangwyn' described 'their' residents as 'high dependency' in that they needed physical care as well as a high level of domestic care. At interview 60 per cent of staff members in 'Brangwyn' said that they spent the majority of their time on domestic tasks. Staff dealt with this by describing their role as that of the care that a nurse would give to children.

On the other hand, in 'Hendy' two of the residents were able physically to engage in a number of domestic tasks. At interview the majority of staff (67%) said that they were engaged in domestic tasks, 33 per cent also said that they socialised with residents and 17 per cent said that they were also involved in rehabilitation. Staff regarded resident home ownership to be an important concept and that they were 'like friends helping residents out in their own homes'. However, observation revealed that instruction and prompting about manners at the table was reminiscent of the parent-teenager relationship.

In contrast, residents in 'Dayspring' were more socially independent. Robert often went out by himself, especially to choir practice, Richard had his own structures in terms of work at the hospital and the local day centre and Howard enjoyed talking and joking with the staff. Robert tended to make decisions for the other two residents and would often answer for Howard. He therefore appeared to be the leader of the three, a kind of older brother. Similarly staff adopted a quasi-sibling role of older brothers and sisters, sometimes chastising their younger kin but also socialising with them. However, at interview, all five staff stated that they saw their position of carer as that of a domestic/housekeeper.

Residents in 'Woodlands' on the other hand were regarded by staff as older relatives. Whilst Timothy was the most active of the three and liked to talk to local shopkeepers and meet friends at the day centre, Sidney and Walter were generally very quiet. All three men also tended to be very slow in their physical functioning. All had a pronounced stoop and took on the appearance of frail elderly people. Staff responded to this by treating them as older relatives, caring for their physical and domestic needs and providing them with company. At interview, 80 per cent of the project workers reported that they perceived their role as carers to be that of a friend whilst only one actually stated that they perceived themselves to be a relative, one a rehabilitation worker and one a nurse. Staff did not expect residents to do much in the way of domestic chores.

Whilst residents in 'Cliffton' were dependent upon staff for domestic care, they were mixed in terms of their social interests. James was very active in both life domains. In particular he was very independent socially and engaged in many activities away from the house. Ruth had difficulties walking and Owain said very little. They usually sat in the lounge for most of the day. Staff tended to adopt an interventionist role for domesticity but left individuals to pursue their separate social interests. Eighty per cent of staff said that they saw their role of carer as a domestic.

Finally, residents in Mountain View were less dependent upon staff for domestic and physical care than their peers in Greentrees. Mountain View was portrayed as a permanent home for those who wanted it but more as a stop-gap, a half-way house to more independent living. The main orientation of Mountain View apart from 'self responsibility' and 'freedom of choice' was therefore rehabilitation with 62 per cent of staff stating that they considered themselves as rehabilitation workers.

However, in Mountain View there was a conflict of interest between wanting residents to be rehabilitated and also allowing them to express freedom of choice. Observation indicated that the majority of staff in Mountain View had a relationship with residents which was generally weak, transient and lacking in intimacy. Staff in Mountain View therefore suffered from role ambiguity. Handy (1993), in his work on organisations, argues that role ambiguity results from uncertainty in the minds of either the focal person or individual or the whole role set as to precisely what their role is at any given time. This results in uncertainty about (a) how one's work is evaluated; (b) the scope for advancement; (c) responsibility and (d) uncertainty about others' expectations of one's performance. Whilst Handy argues that role ambiguity is not necessarily disastrous, for example it can provide opportunities for shaping ones own role, incorporating individuality, he also states that it may lead to role stress, which includes tension, low morale, and communication difficulties.

A key worker system was in operation in which individuals had been charged with the responsibility for the coordination of the rehabilitation plans for particular residents. However, Pilling (1991) argues that the key worker system can be dysfunctional to the resident when key workers form intense, therapeutic relationships which result in a series of short-lived relationships. For some residents key workers were the only members of staff they had contact with on a day to day basis. Residents tended to feel that if they had any problems, they had to wait until their key worker was on duty. This heavy reliance on one member of staff could be dysfunctional and unduly constraining.

An informal key worker system was in operation in Greentrees. At interview, 46 per cent of staff said that they regarded themselves to be informal key workers. Rather than formally designated, key worker relationships tended to develop naturally between staff and residents prompted by the coming together of compatible personalities. Staff rotas which brought people together at particular times often took them into contexts where the playing out of routines led to the establishment of stronger bonds with individuals. With three members of staff on duty it was easier to provide individual attention to each resident. This was advocated and encouraged by management. This provided a ready contrast with the more formal key worker arrangement at Mountain View in which key workers' involvement in particular activities with residents was often dependent upon whether they were on duty or whether particular residents wished to engage in activities. Interviews with residents at Mountain View also revealed that some individuals had difficulties naming their key workers. Similar findings were reported by McGrath (1991). In a study of community mental handicap teams she reported that the existence of a key worker did not always mean that the service user was being visited or knew which worker to contact (ibid, p.74).

The discussion so far has indicated that various roles which staff adopt within their constructed models of care may be 'off the wall' - coming as they do, Mountain View for example, out of thin air rather than from an appreciation of individual needs and wishes. However, they may also be determined by the physical and social characteristics of the individuals, as well as by the tasks which need to be undertaken in order to care for them as exemplified in Greentrees. This ties in with the argument postulated by Pilling (1991) that the roles of team members will largely be determined by the tasks facing them. The present research illustrates that staff do not always adopt the parent/child relationship within the family model as reported in studies of carers of mental illness (Hockey and James, 1988; Bloor et al. 1988; McCourt Perring, 1993) and learning disability (Alaszewski, 1988) but that this model is adapted to include sibling roles as well as laissez-faire and interventionist principles which help staff to make sense of their work. Whether or not residents view care received in the same way remains to be seen and is discussed in Chapters 7, 8 and 9.

Care practices

The descriptions so far have suggested that staff make sense of their jobs by adopting roles within variants of a family model of care. This section now looks at how these particular models of care and notions of kinship guide care practices and how such practices mediate the development of individuals' social networks.

Generally care practices were guided by the overall philosophy of the projects. Whilst recognising the need for residents to make choices about their lives, staff in Greentrees also felt that intervention was necessary. The rationale behind this was that the residents had had decisions made for them for many years whilst in hospital and that it was now difficult for them to make decisions by themselves. Paradoxically, the same logic was used in Mountain View to encourage residents to make decisions about all aspects of their lives.

These differences in decision-making had direct consequences for the development of individuals' social contacts. For example, in 'Hendy' where staff worked within the parental/maternal homely model, all decisions concerning the structure of residents' activities were made by staff, mirroring a parent/child relationship. In terms of rehabilitation and social integration, an emphasis was placed upon good table manners and eating habits within a social skills development framework. Using the adapted Hospital Hospices Practices Profile (HHPP), the rigidity of regime in terms of care practices was found to be of a score of 28 on a scale of 1-53. This was the highest score for all six settings and reflected the researcher's field observations which showed that both residents and staff were involved in well demarcated routine daily tasks. Similarly, 83 per cent of staff reported that there was a regular routine within the house. However, since 'Hendy' was geographically isolated, care was home-based and domestic tasks took up most of the day. As a consequence, there was little time in which to use these social skills. This might explain why the total number of community members (social acquaintances and service contacts) was only one (a service contact) and why the total network membership of residents quantified from resident and staff interviews as well as participant observation data in 'Hendy' was 47, lower than in all but one of the other houses.

Similarly, in 'Dayspring' most decisions about structuring the day were made by staff. They regarded physical presentation to be important within this context and concentrated their domestic tasks to this end, encouraging all three men to wear clean clothes, and to look neat and tidy. Emphasis in this household was placed upon new experiences such as outings to plays, the cinema and a barge holiday - all activities that residents had missed whilst in hospital. These outings were part of a kind of re-living of teenage years. The score for the rigidity of regime using the HHPP in this house was 25, again reflecting a fairly structured care environment, and all 5 staff reported that they worked within a routine each day. Largely as a result of an emphasis on residents' personal presentation and the commitment by staff to take residents to the local community 'Dayspring' residents had the highest total network members (95) of all five houses and the highest total number of community network members (29 social acquaintances and 10 service contacts).

However, in 'Woodlands', social skills and personal presentation were deemed not to be as important as in 'Dayspring'. Care practices were therefore home-based and staff engaged in most domestic activities. The HHPP score was 21 which reflected a less strict regime than the other houses. This was substantiated by staff interviews, four out of five staff reported that there was no routine to the house. Since staff regarded themselves to be surrogate relatives of the residents, community integration was not a priority. The lack of community-based activities for residents due to staff commitment to home based care helps to explain why the total network membership for the residents in 'Woodlands' was 35, lower than that of 'Hendy' and 'Dayspring' where care structures incorporated a commitment to community integration. There were only two service contacts associated with residents in 'Woodlands'.

By contrast there was little routine in 'Cliffton'. The model of care combined interventionism within a laissez-faire approach. The score for rigidity of regime in this house using the HHPP was 23 which was lower than that of 'Hendy', 'Dayspring' and 'Brangwyn' but higher than 'Woodlands'. Again, this was supported by the staff interviews which showed that three out of five staff reported that there was no routine. Although a family atmosphere was identified, the model was less visible than in the other houses. The network score for this house was 74, and included 10 social acquaintances and 22 service contacts. However, the reason for this high score was attributable to one resident, James, who was particularly gregarious, rather than the result of care practices orientated towards social integration.

In 'Brangwyn', the level of rigidity of routine using the HHPP was 24. This was lower than 'Hendy', but higher than the other three houses. All of the staff in 'Brangwyn' stated that there was a routine to which the staff and residents adhered. Care practices in 'Brangwyn' were based around the physical care of two of the residents, within the remit of the maternal/child family model, but there were opportunities for residents to meet others. Staff were very near to Small Market and since one resident, Matthew, was particularly keen to keep active, staff took residents on many excursions and to events where individuals had opportunities to meet new people. This may explain why, despite residents' physical disabilities, the total network membership for this group of individuals was 42, higher than 'Woodlands' where residents did not present as so dependent upon staff. 'Brangwyn' residents also had more contact with community network members (one social acquaintance and four service contacts) than those at 'Woodlands'.

Finally, the HHPP score for Mountain View was only one, some twelve months after the residents had moved in. This low score reflected the laissez-faire philosophy and practice adopted by Mountain View staff in which rigidity of routine was discouraged. All staff also reported that there was no daily routine at the house. There were on average more community members associated with residents in Greentrees than in Mountain View (five and three respectively), illustrating how care practices can both mediate and hinder the development of relationships with members of the community. At Mountain View new social contacts were largely the result of initiatives taken by residents themselves.

Summary

- Each of the community residences had a unique care philosophy and a characteristic way of operationalising that philosophy.
- The laissez-faire philosophy at Mountain View afforded staff considerable autonomy but seemed at the same time to be responsible for confusion or ambivalence among staff about their role and role performance. The key worker system was less than fully implemented.
- Reflecting variants of a family model of care, the philosophy at Greentrees houses was more evidently interventionist. There was greater attention to residents' personal presentation and to their involvement in domestic chores. Daily activities were generally more structured.
- More interventionist care practices, coupled with an emphasis on assisting residents' personal presentation and social skills development, appeared to be helpful in fostering more contacts with community members.
- The significance of these helping behaviours to residents is considered in subsequent chapters.

6 Social networks, social support, social lives - case studies

> An ordinary life is about managing personal relationships, trying to succeed at snooker, worrying about work and money. Painful or not, they are aspects of life which create a sense of self and identity, difference and self-worth.
>
> (Youll and McCourt-Perring, 1993, p.167)

Introduction

Through the presentation of case studies an attempt is made in this chapter to provide a more holistic picture of individuals' social lives, complementing the accounts in Chapters 3 and 4. Descriptions are given of individuals' life histories, including their experiences leading up to and during hospitalisation, and their everyday activities in new community settings. Detailed knowledge of residents' everyday lives is also intended to help to throw some light on how individuals come to attribute meanings to their contacts (Chapter 8) and to discern more precisely the types of social support provided to them through these relationships. A substantial amount of data was generated from the case studies but here we present merely brief vignettes of all 25 residents. The majority of residents in the case study sample were men so the accounts present a predominantly male view of life in the community. Despite the gender imbalance, which would have remained unchanged with any other sampling strategies, it was felt that the accounts of the two women were detailed enough to give a reasonable understanding of the lifestyles of both male and female residents. The descriptions provide a contrast to the life histories by McCourt Perring (1993) which are based purely on the experiences of women.

Findings from the Social Network Interview (SNI) (Chapter 4) about the size and membership of people's social networks are re-evaluated in light of analysis of the case studies. Emergent themes about residents' social lives begin to demonstrate how environmental and historical factors can shape how individuals express themselves. The figures reported about the size and membership of people's social networks in the following vignettes are derived from participant observation methods.

Twenty five case study vignettes

Jane

Jane was born in 1926 and never married. She is a tall woman with a slight stoop. She likes to wear colour co-ordinated clothing. Jane is softly spoken, preferring to speak in her first language - Welsh. Jane is very 'independent'. She cooks for herself and self medicates. She requires little support from project workers at Mountain View apart from encouragement to carry on being 'independent'. Jane tends to be preoccupied with certain subjects such as her own personal hygiene. She enjoys going to jumble sales and cafés, these being her main pastimes. Jane's first admission to the local psychiatric hospital was in 1947 at the age of 21 years. This began a revolving door scenario which included 17 attempts to discharge her into the community. She now feels that Mountain View is her home for life. She lives in a ground floor one bedroomed self-contained flat with adjoining door to the staff kitchen. She had a social network of 32 members comprised mostly of other residents, hospital contacts i.e. staff, though she also had two family members as well as various service providers. Jane seemed to derive mainly physical support, emotional encouragement and company through her social network. Jane has since been transferred to a residential nursing home after a physical illness. Jane says that she likes the residence but misses the independence she had at Mountain View. Her social network has diminished to approximately 12 members.

Daniel

Daniel was born in 1940. He is tall, portly and tends to incline his head. It is difficult to initiate any eye contact with him. Like Jane, he is single, and also likes to converse in Welsh, his first language. Daniel retains his close affinity with his home town and frequently returns there. He has been described by staff as a 'free spirit' since he goes on excursions for days at a time. Daniel has a vivid sense of humour but tends to appear as a 'recluse' as he stays in his flat much of the time. He is a heavy smoker. He was first admitted to Castleton Hospital in 1978. He is on a high dosage of six medications. Seven attempts were made to discharge and re-house Daniel in the community but these proved unsuccessful. Daniel was re-located in Mountain View in November 1990.

The most important member in Daniel's social network is his sister whom he occasionally telephoned and visited. She also sent him money and tobacco. Since Daniel often stays in bed until late afternoon, his interaction with staff and other residents is minimal. Although 11 staff are part of his social network, Daniel feels that only one of them, his key worker, is significant as she speaks Welsh to him. Daniel named eight other residents and participant observation indicated that the exchange of cigarettes was the main function of interactions. Although he shares a first floor flat with Peter there is little communication between them. Daniel has 29 members in his social network. Daniel has since moved into a terraced house in Castleton. He still visits and has stayed at Mountain View, enjoying the company. He has retained the same social network members, making very few new contacts.

Saul

Saul was born in 1944. Like many others in the sample he never married. He has a broad smile. He also tends to cough and splutter due to his heavy smoking habit of 80 cigarettes or more a day. He was admitted to Castleton Hospital in 1966. Before his admission to hospital Saul worked as an electrical fitter. He likes football and played at the hospital. He is on a high dose of medication which includes a fortnightly injection. Saul has had many re-admissions to hospital. Attempts at discharging him to various community settings were proven to be unsuccessful in the past. He rummages in bins for cigarette stubs and spits on the floor. Saul is known as a 'nuisance' and a 'pest and cadger' by staff and other residents. He tends to neglect personal hygiene and could be found walking around Castleton wearing neither a shirt nor shoes. Most of his money is spent on cigarettes. He can invariably be found pacing up and down.

Saul's parents are his only visitors, coming to see him weekly. The rest of Saul's social network comprises residents and staff. Saul has a close affinity to Sarah, a fellow resident. They often chat and tease each other in a jovial way. He also talks a lot to Chris. The two go swimming together. Saul does communicate with the other residents but this tends to be regarding the exchange of cigarettes. Saul has a social network of 29 members. Saul was re-admitted to hospital approximately nine months after his relocation into the community. He is now living in a residential care home in a nearby seaside resort.

Paul

Paul was born in 1941. He is also single. He can often be seen walking half on the pavement, half on the road and intermittently turning round in circles. He can also sometimes be seen praying in public with his hands closed together. He has grown a long beard which he prefers not to cut. He is of a quiet disposition but can be sociable and talkative at times. Paul chain smokes without stopping to flick the ash from the cigarette and the proprietors of a local café often ask him to leave the premises and to return when he has finished his smoke. His first admission to hospital was in 1960, i.e. Paul had spent a total of 29 years in psychiatric hospitals. He has had numerous hospital jobs as an in-patient, working as a printer, in addition to spending time in the industrial therapy unit and occupational therapy unit. Since his relocation at Mountain View, he has joined in the workshop once a week and recently started doing odd jobs around the building such as sweeping the courtyard. The main motivation for these activities appeared to be to gain money for cigarettes.

Paul's social network has a membership of 40. He visits his father and his sister about once a month. Apart from his fellow residents, Paul interacts with individuals he knows from his ward in the hospital. He also knows various shopkeepers in Castleton. Paul is fairly well liked by staff in Mountain View as well as his social worker, community psychiatric nurse and link worker from the local community mental health team. Five years later, Paul now lives in one of the Greentrees houses. His father has since died, but Paul is still in contact with his sister. Paul now has a very active lifestyle and he attends a structured activity every day including two local day centres and an art class. He has shaved off his beard, wears very smart clothing and now smokes his cigarettes much more slowly than he used to. He presents as being very happy. Whilst his network size has shrunk (27 network members) membership has altered somewhat to include rather more fellow residents than staff.

Chris

Chris was born in 1950. He is single and lived with his parents in their own hotel until his first admission to hospital in 1971. He was a very good cricketer at school. He has vivid blue eyes. He is always smiling and is interested in the daily lives of others. Chris will always greet people by name. He is a very popular resident with both staff and residents. Chris has had 16 attempts at resettlement. Chris lives in a single flat situated in the 'cottages' a few yards from the main house. He has skills in cooking, frying, boiling, laundry and ironing. He showers frequently as he states that he is 'magnetised through paper' and that showering relieves this. He frequently has aural hallucinations, delusional ideas, and has a marked tremor of the hand. Chris tends to spend most of his money on cigarettes. Project workers manage his money and give him £2 per day. Chris enjoys being 'independent'. However, he tends to stay in bed until late afternoon if not woken up by a project worker. He occasionally attends the workshop and will go swimming with Saul but most of his day is spent around Mountain View. Chris likes the company of staff, especially when shopping.

Chris was in regular contact with six family members. The rest of his network was comprised of his fellow residents, other ex-patients from the hospital and staff. His network had a total of 39 members. (Chris died of natural causes approximately one year after his relocation into the community.)

Gareth

Gareth is 48 eight years old. He is single, has dark hair and looks young for his age. He left school at 16 years, worked in the local aluminium factory and had various other casual labouring jobs. He was first admitted to Castleton in 1963 at the age of 19 after he had been involved in petty crime and violent behaviour. He was referred by the Magistrates Court but the doctor's report stated 'I felt as though he was a dullard who could best be helped by attempts to find him suitable employment'. However, after sending a threatening letter to his former teacher he was admitted to hospital. In 1964 he was sectioned under the Mental Health Act 1959. He has remained in Castleton Hospital almost continuously since that time. He self-medicates. He dislikes having to do shopping but can and does do some washing and ironing. He is a chain smoker and tends to spend all his money on cigarettes. Staff feel that he reverts to 'psychiatric patient roles' to get what he wants, namely cigarettes or money. Since living at Mountain View, he has carried on working in the gardens of Castleton once a week but spends much of his time wandering the corridors seeing 'old friends'. He has been barred from two public houses in Castleton for verbally abusive behaviour and a local café has complained about his inappropriate sexual advances towards women. Like Saul, he would go round the bins looking for cigarette butts and would supplement his cigarette supply by smoking newspapers. Gareth takes two types of medication which are dispensed to him by staff. Gareth states that he cannot get along with the other residents because they are institutionalised.

Gareth has one sister with whom he is in contact. The rest of Gareth's network (a total of 31 members) comprises staff and residents. At the present time, Gareth no longer works at Castleton Hospital because it has closed. He complains about having nothing productive to do. There has been no significant change in the membership or size of Gareth's social network.

Albert

Albert was born in 1935. He is single. Albert can be found every day sitting in the lounge either reading the newspapers or sleeping. He is careful with his money. He is extremely courteous and gentle. Albert creates humour through his use of puns. He enjoys going to cafés and having tea and a cake. He insists on paying for whoever accompanies him.

Albert is epileptic and had his first seizure at three years of age. He has been on medication since the age of four. He attended a special school until he was seven years old and then lived in an epilepsy 'colony' until he was sixteen years old. He absconded and was then sent to a mental hospital. He has remained in the psychiatric system ever since. He still has grand mals and seizures. Albert has been relocated to a local hostel but this was unsuccessful and he was re-admitted to Castleton Hospital. Staff dispense Albert's medication every day. Albert does not think of himself as a patient and subsequently does not associate himself with the other residents. He tends to mix only with the staff. In particular, he complains about his flat mate. He often attends the workshop.

Albert has five family members who phone him weekly. They have visited him but although he would very much like to visit them, so far they have not encouraged him to do so. Although Albert named all the other residents in Mountain View, he stated that only one was a friend who had been on his ward at the hospital. Albert stated that a service provider, the bank manager, was significant as he received letters from him. These are to do with his bank account. His network has a total of 31 members. Albert has since moved to the same residential care home as Jane. Unfortunately his physical health has deteriorated and he has spent periods of time in hospital. His network is now mostly confined to other fellow residents in the care home.

David

David was born in 1954 and never married. He is tall and has clear blue eyes. He is articulate and likes to have conversations about 1960s music and art. He has aspirations of becoming an artist and has attended various classes. He is also learning French via tapes. David can usually be found in the local cafés as he prefers to eat out rather than cook for himself. He is fond of tea and coffee and will move from one café to the next most days. He smokes rolled cigarettes. David sees Mountain View as a staging post to other accommodation. He feels that taking medication is degrading and he also has difficulty in understanding why he is taking it as he feels that he is not ill. David shares a flat with Albert but there is little communication between them.

David is well liked by the other residents but he tends to socialise more with 'friends' outside of Mountain View as he feels that he cannot relate to the residents as they are all mentally ill. These 'friends' include staff, ex-patients and their families and service providers in Castleton. He has also made friends with a few local people who frequent the local cafés. David finds that he can talk to these individuals about his life, worries and aspirations but apart from visits to the café, he does not do anything else socially with them. David speaks to his mother on the telephone almost every night and visits her most weeks. He also has an aunt and uncle whom he sees about once a month. His network consists of 43 members. The last five years have been eventful for David. He was re-admitted to hospital approximately two and a half years after his relocation into the community. He has been physically ill but has now returned to Mountain View. David now states that he needs medication and that he knows that he will always have to take it. David's social network has remained fairly constant. Individuals have changed, but membership categories have not.

Sarah

Sarah was born in 1942. She is of small stature and has blue eyes. Her clothes are always co-ordinated. She lives in a one person flat which she has furnished herself. It is always spotlessly clean and tidy. She enjoys knitting, sewing and crochet.

Sarah left school at 15 years of age and worked for 12 years in various kitchen or domestic jobs. Her first admission to psychiatric hospital was in 1969 with a depressive disorder and she has had nine admissions since this time. She has been diagnosed as a 'paranoid schizophrenic with active psychosis, deluded hallucinations and emotionally persecutory delusional thoughts'. Sarah self-medicates. Sarah will occasionally join the Mountain View 'workshop' and will also work in the garden but most days she either shops or goes to cafés with friends.

Sarah is prone to bouts of depression when she will cry and not talk to anyone. She also tends to become paranoid at times. Despite these problems, she has a social network of 45 members. Apart from her family, including three siblings, these members are almost entirely staff or other contacts she knows through the psychiatric system. Sarah is known by service providers though this is mainly in connection with paranoid experiences she has had whilst on the premises in the past. Sarah enjoys a particularly friendly relationship with a small core of other residents. Sarah likes to deal only with her key worker regarding her worries, most of which are to do with money. Sarah was re-admitted to Castleton hospital approximately two and a half years after living in the community and has spent short periods of time in the psychiatric unit of the general hospital. She has now returned to her flat in Mountain View. Sarah's life now has slightly more structure than it has done in the past. Her social network has decreased slightly to 41 network members.

Peter

Peter was born in 1939. He is single, tall and burly and has vivid blue eyes. He likes to keep his hair very short. Peter can drive and owns a car. He is a heavy smoker and drinker and usually spends most of his day in the local pub. Peter's psychiatric history has spanned many years beginning in 1964. He has had 22 admissions in all, most of them short stay. Peter has to make sure that he is in Mountain View at midday each day to receive medication from staff. Peter feels that this restricts his social life in that he has to return to the house at specific times. He is always clean and tidy. His employment was in tile laying. He states that he would find it difficult to take work that was poorly paid.

Although Peter's observed social network consists of 23 members, he claims that he is lonely. This is partly due to the fact that he does not wish to be associated with mentally ill persons, and when in ordinary social settings will strive to avoid them by sitting away from them. Peter has had problems with sharing a flat with Daniel who, Peter says '...won't do anything. He's lazy and leaves the kitchen in a mess and he has his radio on late and night and I can't sleep'. Largely due to these problems, Peter has been able to move into a vacant self-contained single flat. He is not in contact with his family by choice as he is self-conscious of living in a residence run by MIND which he feels is degrading. Peter can interact very well on a one-to-one basis and is happy to socialise with a member of staff. He knows very few service providers and he has no social acquaintances. Peter was re-admitted to hospital approximately one and a half years after his relocation into the community. He is now living in Mountain View again. However, he has been quite ill physically and has lost a considerable amount of weight. Peter's social network has not changed significantly in either size or membership.

Thomas

Thomas was born in 1916. He never married. A tall person, he generally says very little and does not usually initiate a conversation but rather tends to speak only when asked questions. Thomas was admitted to Castleton following a mental breakdown aged 26 years and in 1945 he had prefrontal bilateral leucotomy. He was known to stay in bed all day and needed much prompting to do tasks. However, since his arrival at Greentrees, he makes his own breakfast, assists in the weekly shopping and cooks puddings and cakes. He also enjoys gardening and grows tomatoes, lettuce and plants in his greenhouse. Nevertheless, he has to be discouraged from sleeping in the day. He goes horse riding every week. However, he spends much time 'in thought' and, according to case files, 'the overall impression is that Thomas is bored'.

Thomas's social network consists of 15 members. These include his sister and brother who write to him and visit him at least once a year. Apart from the riding instructor, Thomas's only other network members are staff and other residents. There is a marked improvement in Thomas's general demeanour. He is more talkative and not as shy. Thomas's social network now consists of 13 members.

Andrew

Andrew was born in 1933. He is extremely tall and of large build. He did two years' National Service and then went on to study for a degree at university where he participated in football, rugby and athletics. Andrew has retained his love of running and swimming and watching sports on the television. He also enjoys reading and writing and keeps notes in a file about 'the goings on in the house'. Andrew does many of the household chores including the hoovering and gardening. He writes often to his mother. Andrew is a chain smoker and staff restrict this by only allowing him a certain number of cigarettes a day. Consequently, he is always asking if he can 'have me fags'. Andrew tends to talk in monosyllabics and he often laughs to himself as though in a world of his own.

Andrew's social network of 19 members comprises staff and other residents from the other project houses, some of whom he states are his 'friends'. He meets them at the art club which he attends in the town where he has also got to know the art teacher. He visits his mother about once a month and is happy when she gives him sweets and cigarettes. Five years later, Andrew's life is much the same. He presents as having more concentration than before and appears more relaxed. His social network now has approximately 15 members. One previous contact is deceased, and Andrew has not been in contact with three others for an appreciable length of time.

Stephen

Stephen was born in 1920. Like many of his peers who use psychiatric services he never married. He left school at 14 years and worked as a labourer at the local

Colliery. When he was 22 an accident at work left him with head injuries which led to fits and violent outbursts. He was admitted to Castleton in 1962 and then transferred to the sister hospital in 1970 where he resided until he was resettled to 'Hendy' in 1990. He has no surviving family. Stephen is a Welsh speaker. Stephen likes nothing better than to sit in the lounge watching television or listening to the radio. He states that he is retired and does not wish to do any work including household chores. He likes a game of snakes and ladders and will always initiate conversations. Stephen does not smoke. He does not understand money values very well. When he was in hospital he had cataracts on his eyes and was practically blind. Once he moved to 'Hendy', he had an operation to restore eyesight.

Stephen's social network has a membership of 13 people comprised of staff and residents. Stephen says that he is still enjoying living in 'Hendy' and likes to 'take things easy'. He is very happy that he can see more clearly now. His social network has increased slightly in size to 15 members, most of whom are fellow Greentrees residents.

Robert

Robert was born in 1923. He is single, of medium height and large build. Robert left school at 14 years of age and worked at the local colliery. In 1960 he was admitted to Castleton Hospital following violent behaviour. He was diagnosed as suffering from schizophrenia. Robert has had nine admissions to hospital. Since moving to his project house, Robert has been very active. He sings in the church choir, attends art club and the local day centre. Robert is a Welsh speaker. He has an extensive network of 54 members. Apart from fellow residents and staff in the project, Robert has formed relationships with many members of the church choir. Some of them give him a lift home in the car after practice. He has also met individuals from shops and cafés in town. Robert now says that although he still likes his home, 'things are not the same' since his friend and fellow resident, Howard died. Since Howard's death, there have been two consecutive residents living at 'Dayspring', both of whom Robert says are 'OK' but are not really 'his type'. Robert's social network has remained at 54 members despite two previous contacts having since died. This is as a result of his continued involvement with activities outside of the house. Robert states '...it's a good idea to be busy, aye, I'm happier here, yeh, I feel fairly well too, can't complain you know'.

Howard

Howard was born in 1922. He is very tall and like many of the residents he smokes. In 1954 he was admitted to Castleton Hospital diagnosed as having simple schizophrenia as well as being labelled a 'dullard'. He has also had ECT treatment. Howard loves to read and visits the local library every week. He is also very sociable with staff, especially at night when the other residents have retired to bed.

He attends the local church and knows all the words to many hymns off by heart. He loves to sing and to dance.

At the time of fieldwork Howard was in contact with his cousin. Apart from staff and residents, Howard knew only service providers in local cafés, the minister from the church he attended and a few neighbours. He had a total of 12 network members. Howard died during the fieldwork period of natural causes, approximately one year after his relocation into the community.

Richard

Richard was born in 1930. He is very tall, of large build and is single. He was admitted to Castleton Hospital in 1948 following violent behaviour. The same year he had a bilateral prefrontal leucotomy. He has remained in the hospital until moving to his Greentrees project house. In 1972 hospital records referred to him as 'highly institutionalised, post psychotic, and thought-disordered'. Richard has difficulty reading and writing but loves to send post-cards when he goes on holiday as well as Christmas and birthday cards.

Richard has recently renewed contact with his brother whom he writes to and visits. He still works on the hospital gardens and so meets individuals he has known for a long time there including the manager of the gardens. Richard also knows people at the local day centre. Richard's social network totals 27 members. Five years later, he still attends the local day centre and art class. However, whilst he enjoys telling people that he helps around his house, especially with the garden, he still talks about his past 'job' of working in the hospital kitchens. He does not go to church as often as in the past, apparently because there are no staff able to accompany him. His social network now consists of 21 contacts. The closure of Castleton hospital has meant that one social context for Richard is no longer available. The decrease in Richard's network size may be attributed to this factor. Two of his former contacts have also since passed away.

Walter

Walter was born in 1924. He never married. He was in the merchant navy for two years. In 1942 he was admitted to Castleton Hospital at the age of 18 years, and has had several admissions since then. Walter has been described by staff as a 'loveable rogue'. He has a wry sense of humour and when he was in hospital he would joke with patients and staff. Since moving to his new Greentrees home he has become much quieter and normally sits in the lounge all day.

Walter has a small social network of just eight members who are staff and fellow residents. Walter's social network has decreased since he moved to his Greentrees house on account of the fact that he does very little apart from sitting in a chair all day. After a long illness, Walter died of natural causes.

Timothy

Timothy was born in 1920. He is a small, quiet man with a pronounced stoop. He likes to spend time on his own and passes a large part of the day sitting in the garage or garden shed smoking. He is very softly spoken. Since his arrival at his new home, Timothy is less shy and will initiate conversations, something he did not do in the hospital. He likes to do household chores and has a routine for washing up. He is very clean and tidy. He likes to go to the local shop and enjoys meeting acquaintances. He also attends the local day centre.

Timothy has a network of 14 members. He has one brother who comes to visit him. Apart from staff and residents, Timothy has also formed a relationship with two local shopkeepers. Since the original fieldwork was undertaken Timothy has suffered a physical illness which left him unsteady on his feet. He is now semi-dependent on a wheelchair. Despite this or, as staff claim, 'because of this', Timothy is much more talkative than previously and smiles more. It is noticeable that he receives more attention from staff than before due to his increased physical dependency. He states that he likes to go out and about when the staff will take him but that he still likes to dry the dishes when he can. On the other hand, he says that he misses Walter who used to live in the same house. He gets on less well with the new person who has replaced Walter. Timothy's social network remains at 14 members with two shopkeepers being replaced by two other residents.

Sidney

Sidney was born in 1927 and never married. He is of medium height and is always smartly dressed. Sidney smokes heavily. He walks at a slow pace with his head inclined. Sidney was first admitted to hospital in 1953 and has spent 31 years there. He is in contact with his brothers who visit him once a fortnight. They bring him cigarettes and take him for rides in the car. Sidney has an interest in cars and used to own a motor cycle when he was younger.

Sidney's social network consists of his four family members, a number of staff members and fellow residents. They constitute a social network of 13 members. At the time of fieldwork, Sidney had to return to hospital for a brief spell as he became ill. Sidney is now back at his home, his life very much the same as it was five years ago. He is more talkative than previously and again smiles more but says that he doesn't do much 'cos I've got no money'. He now has ten members in his social network. One previous contact has died and the other two persons, both staff members, have not been in contact with Sidney for an appreciable length of time.

Ruth

Ruth was born in 1932. She is a small woman and likes to talk. She will initiate conversations with most people though the subject is most often about her past life. Ruth spent 24 years in an epileptic 'colony' and was transferred to Castleton

Hospital in 1956. She was diagnosed as being a 'simple, childish woman with epileptic psychosis and borderline subnormality'. She has later been diagnosed as having chronic schizophrenia. Ruth tends to sit in the lounge most of the day watching television. Apart from staff and fellow residents, Ruth interacts with her dentist and looks forward to seeing him. She also has an affinity to the families of staff members. Her social network comprises 16 members. At the present time Ruth describes herself to be 'quite happy' with her life and the way the house is run. Her own social network now has 14 members.

James

James was born in 1912. He was married but all contact with his wife has been severed. He is a small man with a pronounced stoop. Friendly and talkative, he walks with his head forward and his arms behind his back. James is very active for his age. He likes to lay the table for meals and will do other household chores such as taking the bins out and paying the milkman. James is busy most days. He attends the local day centre twice a week, the art club, and goes on various excursions run by MIND. He collects post-cards and keeps an account on paper of everywhere he has been. James knows many people. At the time of fieldwork, he had formed a close relationship with a woman he met at the day centre. There were 46 people in his network. All of the members in James's social network have associations with the hospital. James has recently become a little confused and has been known to wander onto the busy main road by his house. He cannot walk long distances and becomes frustrated because he is not so independent as he used to be. Three of James's previous contacts have died and people he once knew, such as the milkman and taxi man, have now been replaced by other individuals he knows less well. Despite this, his social network now consists of 44 members though they consist almost entirely of staff and other residents, hospital contacts, with only one additional social acquaintance whom he met at his local chapel.

Owain

Owain was born in 1930 and is a Welsh speaker. He will only speak when prompted and usually answers in one or two words. He is slightly deaf. He was brought up on a farm in rural Wales until his admission to Castleton Hospital in 1947 when he was aged 17 years. He remained there until leaving in 1990 for his new Greentrees home. He was diagnosed as being mute with schizoid behaviour. Owain is very solitary and communicates with a nod of his head or by pointing. However, since moving to his new home, he has begun to use short sentences to make his wishes known. His appearance is neat and tidy. He does little else apart from sitting in the lounge watching television for most of the day. Owain has 15 members in his network who include staff and their relatives and other residents. Since the research was first carried out, Owain smiles more and will say a few more words but still remains shy, quiet and tends to sit in the house lounge for most of the day. His social network now consists of 12 members.

Frederick

Frederick was born in 1916 and has never been married. When he was five years old he fell down some stairs and fractured his skull. This may have resulted in his learning difficulties as he left school at 14 years, able only to write his name. He has very poor eyesight but loves to be outdoors. He is a naturist and likes to sunbathe in the nude. Frederick was a fitter for a company for 12 years. His first admission to psychiatric hospital was in 1945. A year later he lost his employment. In 1957 he was readmitted with fits of temper and aggression. He was later admitted to Castleton Hospital in 1974. Frederick has nine members in his social network who are fellow residents and staff. Five years later Frederick has had an operation to remove a cataract from his eye. He presents as weak and frail but still retains his sense of humour. His social network has not changed in size, though his former co-resident, Edward, has been replaced by another, Paul.

Matthew

Matthew was born in 1920. He is an only child and has never been married. He had one job as a messenger boy for a local grocery store. Matthew is small, stoops and tends to lower his head when communicating. He has a soft voice and likes to joke. Matthew spent 46 years in Castleton and its sister hospital. Matthew likes to accumulate items such as clothes and shoes. He also has to be supervised and prompted about his personal hygiene. Matthew is a keen horse rider and attends the riding club every week. He is driven there by a member of staff. He also goes to art class and attends chapel. He is a heavy smoker and staff restrict him to one 'light' per hour because of his smoker's cough. Matthew has a social network of ten people who are either staff or residents. He proudly shows off his recently awarded rosette for achievement at horse riding. Matthew continues to be witty, happy and friendly although he misses Edward who died recently. Matthew's social network has not changed in size in the last five years, although Edward has been replaced by Paul, whom Matthew says he can 'have a laugh' with.

Edward

Edward was born in 1919. He is single and a Welsh speaker. He was regarded as a shy boy and considered himself to be a ci bach (underdog). He left school at 15 years old and became a farm worker. In 1958 he was admitted to a psychiatric hospital in the South of England. He was admitted to Castleton in 1962 and diagnosed as a paranoid schizophrenic. Edward is well known in Small Market and walks into town most days. He chats to various people but has had problems with school children who taunt him. Edward tends to stand out as he likes to wear outlandish clothes and a cowboy hat. He can become quite aggressive when this happens and runs after people with a stick. Despite knowing many people in town, Edward's social network is also comprised of staff and residents. He is in contact with his brother and three other family members. He has 23 network members. Edward recently died of natural causes.

The rest of this chapter begins with a re-evaluation of the size and membership of people's social networks by drawing together interview and participation observation data. This is followed by a review of recurrent themes derived from the case studies.

Network size and membership - a re-evaluation

One of the most striking findings drawn from the case studies was the difference in network size between data collected using the SNI and that of participant observation. Apart from participating in residents' everyday lives within their homes, the fieldworker observed individuals' social lives, including their relations with people in local communities. This meant that names provided by individuals during the SNI could be checked and that further network members could be added. The same criterion period of one year was used as well as the same membership categories as for the SNI. The Ethnograph computer programme was used to manage the data, and further network members were coded onto a recording matrix.

Figure 6.1 shows a marked increase in total network size, this difference being highly significant using the Wilcoxon sign test ($p<.0001$). Ethnographic methods revealed that the average network size for all residents was 25, representing nearly double the number found from the SNI schedule. The range of network size also increased from between 2-46 to 8-54. Interestingly, these results are closer to findings relating to well people. Pattison et al. (1975) found that well individuals were able to recall 22-25 people in their network perceived to be important to them. However, since network size in the present study was calculated on the basis of all network members regardless of their perceived importance, study group members appear to have social networks which are still smaller in size than those of general population samples. Nevertheless, the average increase of 12 network members using participant observation methods indicates that the latter method is more likely to gain a fuller picture of total network size than interview schedules alone.

Analysis of these differences by network membership is a little more diagnostic. Participant observation demonstrated that for the whole sample the number of family members increased from 1.8 to 2.2 persons. Three individuals in Mountain View and one in Greentrees were found to have more family members than had been originally stated at interview. Sarah did not mention her brother-in-law at interview, but subsequent conversations revealed that she was in contact with him. This exemplifies the point that interviews are very situational and can be mood specific. When Sarah was feeling 'ill' or paranoid on a particular day, the interview schedules were inappropriate, inefficient and, so far as Sarah was concerned, intrusive. However, on such a day during fieldwork when Sarah was feeling 'down and depressed', the fieldworker took her to a local café where she responded by sharing her life story with the researcher for approximately two hours.

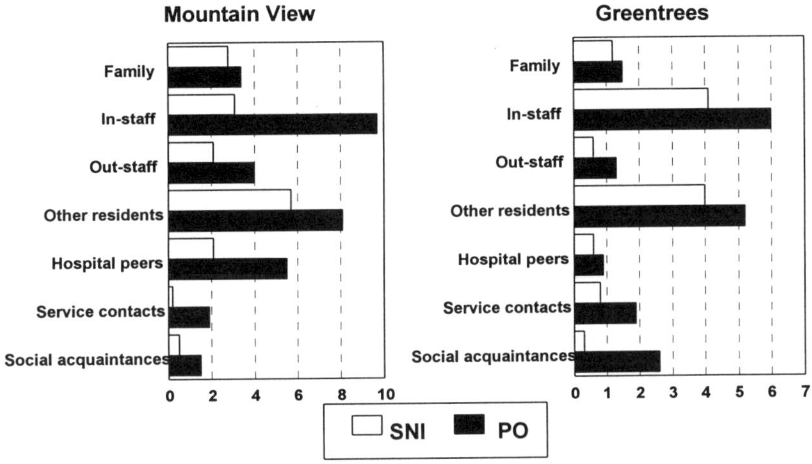

Figure 6.1 Comparison of network size and membership of residents in Mountain View and Greentrees Using two methods - Social Network Interview (SNI) and Participant Observation (Po). (Mean Scores)

There was also a significant increase in the average number of staff members (an average total increase of three in-staff and one out-staff). This was most noticeable in Mountain View where the average number of in-staff increased from three to ten. It was found that individuals had difficulty remembering staff members' names and would tend only to mention those on duty at that particular time but would name the others during more casual conversations. Drugs which deplete concentration may have been a factor here.

An increase was also found in the categories of 'other residents' and 'hospital peers' (4.7 to 6.4 and 1.2 to 2.8 respectively). In all of the categories mentioned so far, data gained from participant observation showed that Mountain View residents had more network members than individuals in Greentrees. However, this was not the case for network scores in the membership category of service contacts. There was an overall increase (0.6 to 1.9) for the study group. Many service contacts observed in cafés and public houses had not been reported by residents at interview. It was interesting to note that whereas the SNI had shown more service contacts for those in Greentrees than in Mountain View (0.8 and 0.2 respectively) observations showed Greentrees residents to have equal amounts of service contacts in their networks as those in Mountain View (1.9).

On the other hand, there was a change in average scores for social acquaintances. Whereas SNI scores showed a slightly larger number of social acquaintances in Mountain View than in Greentrees (0.5 and 0.3 respectively) the position was reversed using data obtained from participant observation. This appeared to be linked to the more structured environment of Greentrees which was committed to helping residents to foster contacts with community members. Although there was also an increase in the range of social acquaintances (0-4 to 0-25), this averaged out at only two social acquaintances per person, indicating that residents are still relatively devoid of such relationships.

It may therefore be argued that quantitative methods only delineate a fraction of the actual total network members. As discussed in Chapter 3, some individuals in the present study had problems communicating. They also found structured interviews tiresome. It might further be argued that previous quantitative methods (Hammer et al. 1978; Sokolovsky and Cohen, 1981; Leff et al. 1990; Dunn et al. 1990 and Anderson et al. 1993) may not be a reliable or appropriate method for gaining information about network size and membership for individuals typical of those in this study. The argument is not one of dismissal of quantitative methods. Wenger (1994) has been successful in measuring the network size and network type of population samples of elderly people. Choice of method appears therefore to be more a question of suitability, with no single method necessarily being right for all individuals. Rather, the lives of different groups of the population who live in different situations and have different problems need to be explored using the most appropriate methods. In the present study participant observation appears to provide a more reliable and comprehensive picture of the social lives of individuals with long-term mental illness than quantitative methods alone.

Recurrent themes

The vignettes above illustrate the individuality of residents as people with distinct personalities, life histories and lifestyles. They highlight the significance of people and events in their lives prior to first admission to hospital which in most cases was decades ago. For example, Saul also talked about his days as an electrical fitter and Timothy recounted helping his parents in their sweet shop whilst Chris talked extensively most days about his role as a cricketer as though it were in the immediate past rather than 20 years or so ago.

However, movement back into the community did not, for most individuals, result in a return to previous roles considered important by them. The only exception was Robert who returned to his former role as a member of a church choir.

For the remainder of the study group, the anonymity of hospital institutional life tended to conceal their former identities as ordinary people, much as other studies had shown (Goffman, 1961; Barham and Hayward, 1991). Unlike the life histories presented by McCourt Perring (1993), these case studies indicated that residents on the whole still identified themselves with the hospital. This was evident in conversations observed between residents and accounts given to the fieldworker in which individuals liked to recount 'old times' at the hospital. Former, almost forgotten roles show glimpses of residents as ordinary people as well as indicating their achievements in different social roles. According to Butler and Rosenthal (1985, p.38) to rehabilitate means to restore a person's physical and mental capacities and improve their quality of life to a level which is as near as possible identical to that which existed prior to illness. Acknowledgement by staff of such previous roles may be one step towards this restoration as well as possible re-establishment of old network members and renewed confidence to develop new social relationships. However, despite changes in social role and community living milieu, one significant part of the study group's lives remained constant, that of the taking of medication.

Medication

Medication has been reported before as forming an important and prominent part of the lives of people with a mental illness (Estroff, 1985). As stated in Chapter 3, the majority of the study group were drug-dependent and 17 were dependent upon staff for the provision and regulation of medication, leaving only 6 out of 25 residents able to self-medicate, and 2 individuals on no medication.

At Mountain View, the administering of medication by staff to residents was the only visible structure imposed on people's everyday lives. This normally took place in the staff kitchen where the medicine cabinet was located. At certain times of the day, particularly early morning, and at meal times, residents would hover around the communal lounge or reception area, waiting for staff to take them to the otherwise locked medicine box.

Medications represent one of the most striking and distinct aspects of the psychiatric world, both among users and non users (Estroff, 1985). During fieldwork a new medical jargon had to be learned in order to understand what staff and residents were referring to when they discussed medications. It was found that medication denotes to the person taking it and to those observing that the person is still ill or dependent in some way. Hospital confinement and patienthood also represent illness whereas hospital discharge is held to represent improved health (Simic, 1994). The hospital as well as psychiatric medicine therefore symbolised mental illness for the residents in this study. Having to take medicine was looked upon by some individuals as a contradiction since their movement into the community was equated with improved health and well-being. This is illustrated by Ruth from Greentrees:

> I live in the community and I'm supposed to be off drugs now. I don't wish to be a drug addict. I told the doctor that too. He asked me 'What do you do with your day?' I told him I sit quietly and behave and so I don't want to be on drugs.

David and Peter, both from Mountain View, felt strongly that people on medication were ill. David stated that he could not communicate with many of the other residents as they were 'drugged up and all out of their heads'. This raises issues about the effects of medication on the social lives of individuals.

Barham and Hayward (1991) found that most of their study group did not mind taking medication, but many felt that incorrect doses could impair their sociability. In the present study, whilst individuals were generally dissatisfied with the type or dose of their medication, no one in Greentrees and few residents in Mountain View stated that the medication actually restricted their social lives. On the other hand, however, observations indicated that residents who had to return to Mountain View at particular times of the day to take medication were reticent to engage in local activities if they thought that they might not be able to return in time for their drugs.

The cigarette sub-culture

Although 40 per cent of the British population over 16 years old smoke (Willis, 1989), as with medication, smoking appears to be a particular feature of psychiatric illness and the majority of residents (19/25) smoked. Fifteen were chain smokers. It was revealed that the majority of the smokers started when they were admitted to hospital.

Observations indicated that the 'cigarette business' was commonplace on the hospital wards, corridors and in particular the coffee bar, a domain not frequented by the staff. This was reminiscent of the TAPS study findings (Dunn et al. 1990). Similar behaviour carried over to Mountain View. However, compared to the hospital wards, smoking appeared to take on an even more important role in the lives of some individuals as at Mountain View there was little other formal structure to their day apart from that offered by medication times. It was found, therefore, that some individuals structured their lives almost entirely around smoking. This is illustrated by Saul, recounting his actions the previous day:

Saul: I got up at 10 past 6 a.m. I went to the office for me money for cigs. I made breakfast myself and had it on my own. At 8 o'clock I had my first smoke and I had a wash and put some clothes on. Then at 11 o'clock I had my second smoke... I go to the swimming baths on a Tuesday and Friday night from 6-7 p.m. then at 7 p.m. I come back to get my cigs.... I borrow cigs from Paul. David shares a cigarette as well, you know.

Thus, for some residents, smoking serves to add an element of organisation to their day. With Mountain View being organised along laissez-faire principles restrictions on cigarettes were not in operation. Although this meant that individuals were able to exercise more autonomy than had been their experience at the hospital, it was not always exactly what they wished. For example, Saul was known for his bouts of coughing and spluttering as well as spitting phlegm - symptoms of years of smoking. He also blamed his outbursts of temper on his smoking habits.

However, at Greentrees chain smokers were viewed as being hazardous to themselves and others. They were therefore only allowed a limited number of cigarettes or lights per day. Again this formed a structure to their day but it was imposed rather than self-imposed. Staff at Greentrees also expected residents to perform certain tasks such as domestic chores before they had their next cigarette and therefore whilst smoking came to be associated with reward for having completed tasks, it did not interfere with any other activities in which they might be engaged. Cigarettes were the main and sometimes only source of conversation between residents.

As will be discussed in the next chapter, the exchange of cigarettes between residents tended to denote friendship. It could also signify an exploitative relationship. It was also a route towards developing relationships in the community.

Poverty

Desperation could also often lead to agitation and confrontation between residents and others. Squabbles between individuals were normally concerned with one resident pestering another for a cigarette. Whilst the negative aspects of the smoking habit such as begging for cigarettes, smoking newspaper, coughing and spitting phlegm are visible to 'outsiders', for some residents cigarette exchange provided a topic for conversation, an expression of friendship and, in some instances, a route towards new network members. At Mountain View in particular there were few other available activities for residents. The culture of smoking and the behaviour associated with it was accordingly likely to remain an important part of residents' lives.

On the other hand, smoking was inextricably linked to poverty. Many residents were reduced to begging from each other as well as staff in efforts to satisfy their craving. On one occasion, for example, Gareth asked a project worker if she could find him something to do for money for a cigarette as he was 'desperate'. She allowed him to clean her car for £1. Working for money to pay for cigarettes, although not usually as blatant as this, was nonetheless common within Mountain View. Gareth, Chris and Paul worked in the workshop at Mountain View solely to earn money for cigarettes. Paul would also sometimes brush the yard or perform other odd jobs for £1 an hour for his 'cigs'. Gareth was also observed to wander around the communal bins in the lounge as well as waste bins in the neighbourhood looking for cigarette stubs. When Saul became desperate, he was observed to smoke newspaper or any rubbish he could find.

All of the residents were in receipt of welfare benefits. At the time of fieldwork, after paying for their rent and food, they had approximately £11 to spend on themselves. For most individuals this meant that they were limited both in real and perceived terms from participating in normative social activities (such as shopping for clothes, luxury items, cinema and theatre outings and so on). Almost all reported that they had 'financial problems'.

Residents like Daniel and David also received a little money from their relatives, but since many individuals' families were either deceased or had lost touch, this potential source of financial support was closed to them.

Some residents managed to earn a little extra money from paid work. Albert, Paul, Chris and Gareth worked in the Mountain View workshop for £1 per hour, as well as doing odd jobs such as sweeping the yard and weeding the garden. However, the workshop was only opened twice a week (Tuesdays and Thursdays). Whilst residents could work as many hours as they wanted on these days, they tended from choice to work only one or two hours at most. Lack of concentration and the craving for cigarettes appeared to be the principal reasons for this short working span. Supplementary income from this source was, therefore, minimal and soon spent.

Although it was found that many residents at Mountain View were prepared to become employed, they were impeded from gaining employment because of restrictions on earnings by the Department of Social Security (DSS). At the time of fieldwork, residents were only allowed to earn approximately £15 per week. This dilemma was very real to Peter:

> I'm restricted. I'm only allowed to earn so much money per week. I tell you what, I haven't half spent some money. I'm getting a bit short now so I need a job. I'd love to have a job now, so many hours, maybe a few quid a week to put back into it again because I've lost me eh, me eh craftsman's skill and everything. I've lost all that.... I'm getting fed up without my car because I can't get the money to spend on it, do you know what I mean? Yeh, I'm skint now, I'm getting skint now....

This quote illustrates the spiral of poverty so common for individuals with a mental illness. Relative poverty for most residents also meant exclusion from social spheres where they may have made new contacts. In particular, residents such as Albert and Gareth felt that community social activities were beyond their reach financially:

Albert: I tried to go to the snooker club, but they were charging £8 to get in so I went off that idea.

Gareth: I don't go for a pint cos I've no money.

Similar findings about the social exclusion effects of poverty were recorded by Barham and Hayward (1991) who argued that 'the social horizons of people, and how they felt about themselves and their prospects, were markedly affected by the limited means at their disposal' (ibid, p.27).

A further factor exacerbating poverty was the lack of budgeting skills, especially for residents at Mountain View. Protracted periods spent in hospital, where personal monies were mostly managed by staff, meant that the responsibility of budgeting could be a difficult task. At Mountain View, residents were expected to budget for themselves with some help from staff. This proved difficult for the smokers who, tending to spend most of their money on cigarettes, would often not have enough money for food.

On the other hand, staff at Greentrees took responsibility for residents' monies and gave them 'pocket money'. This worked well for some residents such as Stephen who stated:

Stephen: I have enough money. They keep it. They gave me £3 yesterday. I just get it now and again. They keep it and it's alright.

For others like James, this was not so satisfactory:

James: When I was in hospital, I used to walk down to Small Market and back and put my money in the Post Office. But I don't get any money here at all. The pension which I sign for - they put that in the bank - TSB or something. But I'd rather have the money to put in the Post Office you know.

R: Have you asked them if you can do that?

James: Oh, no I haven't, no because they come to me and say 'sign the pension book' and they put the money in the TSB and that's all there is to it. I didn't have any say in it you know. I get the odd 50p for today and that's all.

Poverty was therefore a very real phenomenon for residents in the study group and a characteristic that contributed to the loss of opportunities to form new relationships with community members. This however needs to be seen in the context of how individuals generally spent their time.

Use of time

Social relationships which provide supportive functions may only be maintained by spending time with others. Thus the ways in which individuals spend their time is very important. The concept of time and its use has been found to have a different meaning for those living within psychiatric care residences compared to most other persons (Estroff, 1985). Reasons for this relate to employment, poverty, and most significantly, care practices.

It has already been argued that due to a combination of age, illness, medication side effects and DSS restrictions, few residents were or had been employed. The effects of unemployment have been reported to include the marginalisation of some members of society (Lea and Young, 1984), physical and mental ill health, as well as attempted and actual suicide (Allen and Watson, 1986; Laurance, 1986). Exacerbated by problems associated with their illness, the study group are in a difficult situation.

The working environment is also a source of relationships outside of the home. Unemployment therefore represented a route lost to social contacts (Fagin and Little, 1984). The social milieux within which residents moved therefore was made up almost entirely of staff and other residents, hence the findings of social network membership which showed that staff and other residents made up the highest percentage of network members for residents in both projects. These were also the contacts seen the most frequently (daily) by residents.

Since there was a high staff-resident ratio in both Mountain View and Greentrees (1-1 and 5-3 respectively) it followed that a large part of residents' time was spent with staff. So what exactly did individuals do with their time?

The only activities with routines and structures approximating paid work in which individuals in Greentrees were engaged were leisure activities at the craft centre, day centre and horse-riding complex. These had been initiated by the managers. There was also an unwritten rule of compulsory attendance attached to them. Whilst these activities provided structure to individual's lives, for 20/25 residents in the study no distinction was made between work and leisure. Two-thirds of residents spent much of their time sitting, either alone or with another, in silence, watching television, and in addition, 13 of these residents also smoked. Activities such as these could be described as passive (Cotterill, 1994). The following extracts from fieldnotes typify the atmosphere of this situation:

Fieldnotes. 'Cliffton' 17 August 1991

> This afternoon, the house was very quiet. James sat in the front room staring out of the window whilst Owain sat in the back room. He had the television on loud but was not watching it.

Fieldnotes. 'Woodlands' 27 February 1991

> For the duration of my interview with the project worker, Timothy sat outside in the garage smoking whilst Sidney sat in the dining room, silently smoking. Walter sat in the lounge slumped in his seat sleeping, although the television was on.

The other nine residents either had work or activities arranged for them. In Greentrees, days were marked by medication doses, meal times and for many, cleaning and washing up. However, at Mountain View, residents were expected to provide their own meals and clean their own flats, but with no-one to tell residents to do these chores these were very often left undone. Residents tended to eat cold meals which needed little preparation or else they opted to eat out in cafés.

However, since there was little else to do in Mountain View save the few organised workshop days every week, it was none too surprising that residents did very little.

Most Mountain View residents spent much of their day, like many unemployed people, watching television (Kelvin and Jarrett, 1985). Few residents had hobbies with which to punctuate the day and therefore time as a concept had very little meaning to them. Few residents wore watches or asked for the time, one of the reasons why many arrived late to meetings or events. Howe (1995) argues that schizophrenics need stimulation such as structured activities as well as short periods of rest 'to offset the undermining apathy and lethargy of the illness'.

Qualitative data therefore helped to reveal how the ways in which residents spent their time were mediated by historical, structural and personal factors. Individuals were confined to only a few social contexts in which to form new social relationships. Nevertheless, even when individuals did have opportunities to spend time outside of their own residences, personal presentation and communication deficits could also act as barriers to the extension of their social networks.

Personal presentation and communication

The importance of personal presentation to social acceptance or rejection has been well documented (Beels, 1981; Hampson et al. 1984; Bellack and Mueser, 1986). It has been argued that successful transition into the community is mediated by self-maintenance skills such as care of clothes, money management and cooking abilities (Presley et al. 1982). For the residents in this study, an adapted personal presentation checklist (Hampson et al. 1984) was used to present a general picture of what kinds of behavioural traits might preclude individuals' social integration. The results are presented in Table 6.1.

Mountain View residents were more likely to have unusual traits concerning clothes and general appearance than those in Greentrees. In particular, personal hygiene, maintenance of clothing and wearing clothes properly were problematic for them. The reason for this difference lay in the care practices of the two projects. Residents in Greentrees were generally provided by staff with clean clothes on a daily basis. Personal presentation of the residents in all five houses was generally extremely good. However, in Mountain View, an insistence upon residents' rights to freedom of choice meant that to a large extent, if individuals wished to wear dirty and inappropriate clothes, this was their prerogative. Since it has been found that the deterioration in personal hygiene common in schizophrenic patients may predispose them to social rejection even after they have developed inter-personal skills (Bellack and Mueser, 1986) this ought to be an important consideration in community care programmes.

Table 6.1
Personal presentation checklist
Adapted from Hampson, Judge and Renshaw (1984)

Question: *Is there anything unusual about the residents?*

	Mountain View	Greentrees	Total
Clothes			
Cleanliness	4	3	7
Suitability	1	1	2
Maintenance	4	3	7
Put on properly	4	1	5
General			
Face	0	1	1
Hair	2	0	2
Hands	5	3	8
Glasses and teeth	1	1	2
Smell	0	1	1
Eyes	0	2	2
Posture			
Head hangs down	3	10	13
Stomach sticks out - due to posture	3	8	11
Shoulders slumped forward and back bent	7	12	19
Walks with toes in or toes out	0	1	1
Walks with feet apart	1	1	2
Unusual walk, large strides	1	2	3
Are there any unusual traits?			
Dribbling	0	2	2
Very loud talking	4	3	7
Sticking tongue out	0	3	3
Rocking	0	0	0
Movement - leg up and down	7	1	8
Talks in monosyllabics/speech difficult to understand	1	10	11

Scores for each individual
Yes = 1
No = 0

Posture also appeared to be a key feature which might affect the response of local people. Thirteen individuals hung their heads and nineteen slumped their shoulders forward and had a pronounced stoop. Eye contact with these individuals was therefore difficult.

Coupled with this was the fact that 11 residents also either spoke in monosyllables or had incoherent speech. It was therefore difficult to hold conversations with them. This is consistent with other research findings in which poverty of speech was found to be a prominent feature of the negative symptom construct in schizophrenia (Ragin et al. 1989). Similarly, Bellack et al. (1990) found that people with schizophrenia have pronounced deficits in social competence. They were substantially impaired in verbal, non-verbal and overall ratings of social skills as well as in interview ratings of role functioning. Observations of the individuals in this study showed quite clearly that these characteristics were significant to the social integration process. The following extract from a field diary is just one of many examples which illustrate the problems faced by residents due to their own social functioning deficits:

26 June 1991:

As soon as we arrive at Harlech, David states 'I'm suffering from withdrawal symptoms for a cup of tea.' We all laugh. Albert and Saul immediately go to find a lavatory. Saul asks a passer-by in the street stating:

Saul:	Where's the toilet please?
Woman:	What? (looks strangely at Saul)
Saul:	Toilet
Woman:	Speak clearer (getting agitated)
Saul:	Toilet (shouting)
Woman:	Oh round there (she looks in disgust and hurries on)

This extract well illustrates the difficulties for those individuals who have social functioning problems.

Summary

- Methodologically, in studies of the social lives of people with long term mental illnesses participant observation appears to provide a more rigorous, valid and reliable means of data collection than structured interview schedules.

- Participant observation showed that residents in Mountain View had larger social networks than those in Greentrees. However, in terms of network membership, Greentrees residents were found by comparison to have rather more community members in their networks.
- Residents' lives were characterised by experiences which are part of and in most cases consequences of the social problem of mental illness. These include the legacy of hospitalisation, side effects of medication, poverty, chain-smoking, unemployment and a lack of social contexts in which to spend time and form new relationships.
- A lack of structure surrounding patterns of everyday living left some residents, mostly those at Mountain View, with responsibility for setting that structure themselves. There were few signs that this was accomplished.
- Residents were found to be devoid of meaningful 'life roles' in which they could express their identities and self-worth.
- Unlike the women in McCourt Perring's study, who expressed their lives before hospitalisation as including roles within the home, family and work, the vignettes provide a predominately male perspective. They show men entering the psychiatric system at an early age when they had experienced few other social roles. Only two out of twenty three had ever been married and many had never had employment before hospitalisation.
- These men were, therefore, devoid of any immediate family of their own apart from perhaps siblings and, therefore, they have little to talk about apart from life in hospital. This is in complete contrast to the women in McCourt Perring's (1993) study who had relatively little to say about life in hospital, reflecting its low value for them.
- Ways in which the above problems acted as barriers to the development of social networks were also noted. Personal, historical and structural factors were all implicated.

The experiences of individuals and views about social networks and support are the subject of more detailed analysis in the next two chapters.

7 Encountering support - analysing the experience of residents

> Traditional individual - and network - level approaches to the study of social support fail to fully embrace the importance of *meaning* within the social support process.
>
> (Miller and Ray, 1994, p.225)

The aim of the present chapter is to explore more fully how residents experienced support. The constituents of support are not easily separated from relationships and in previous studies these have not always been discussed as different dimensions. It is hoped that a separate analysis of both concepts will provide clues as to the relationship between the two. An analysis of residents' perceptions of their relationships is described in the next chapter. Here we attempt to identify dimensions of support and what meanings they had for individuals.

Descriptions of support in the literature

The literature review in Chapter 1 highlighted the conceptual confusion surrounding the term social support. Kahn and Antonucci (1980) argue that the term social support carries colloquial meaning and has therefore been used more often than defined (ibid, p.267).

One of the reasons for such a diversity of categories within typologies may be because conceptualisations of support have been situation specific. For example, Commerford and Reznikoff (1996), studying nursing home residents, looked specifically at perceived support, information and feedback from family and friends, linking this to the religiosity of residents. On the other hand, Orr et al. (1995) measured eight types of support by drawing upon affective and instrumental categories in a study of people with physical disabilities, linking these to individuals' tendency to conform.

The sheer diversity of categories has been accompanied by a range of meanings and operationalisations. For example, 'instrumental' support was defined by Pattison (1977) to mean mutual aid and financial assistance, but 'aid' was used by House (1981) in terms of money, labour, time and modifying environment. Kempen and Eijk (1995), measuring social support of elderly people, refer to instrumental support along with informative and emotional support in times of trouble as 'support in a problem situation'. On the other hand, Bowers (1987) defined instrumental support as actually 'doing for' residents. Instrumental support such as financial aid has been categorised by others as material aid (Barrera and Ainlay, 1983), aid (Kahn and Antonucci, 1980), and tangible assistance (Cobb, 1979; Richman et al. 1993).

In an attempt to clarify conceptualisations of social support some writers (House, 1981; Barrera and Ainlay, 1983; Richman et al. 1993) have organised the points of confluence within existing taxonomies into what they would describe as more rational typologies of support functions. For example, following a content analysis of literature, House (1981) emerged with what he considered to be the most important support types (emotional, instrumental, informational and appraisal). Indeed, emotional support does appear to be part of many support typologies (see Kempen and Eijk, 1995) as does the provision of practical assistance.

Whilst typologies have been numerous, few were found to have been empirically driven (see Brim, 1974; Gottlieb, 1978). Rather, most were found to be a priori theoretical schemes derived from literature searches of previous taxonomies and adapted for the social group under investigation (see Barrera and Ainlay, 1983; Cohen et al. 1985; Richman et al. 1993). None of the foregoing relate specifically to ex-long-stay psychiatric patients now living in community settings. Furthermore, few support taxonomies were found to map support provided by formal sources.

Nevertheless, typologies grounded in the everyday experiences of the recipients of care are regarded as critical to counter previous typologies based upon highly subjective judgements (Barrera and Ainlay, 1983, p.137). Furthermore, whilst theoretical and operational definitions of social support are abundant, empirical demonstrations of those features of social relationships which are significant in relationship to health, illness (McFarlane et al. 1984) and social integration are lacking.

House (1981) illustrates the difficulties of support typologies by using the example of Huckleberry Finn who received help from Tom Sawyer, the widow Douglas, and his black companion, Jim, but the kinds of support received from each of them were quite different, as were the consequences. House asks what are the differences which make a difference? That is, how many types or forms of social support must be distinguished that have distinctive and important effects for the people under investigation (ibid, p.14)? This leads to a consideration of how recipients of support talk about support.

Identifying types of support

In keeping with the grounded theory approach adopted in Chapter 6 in which characteristics of residents' lives were drawn from the data, support types were identified from the accounts of residents themselves. This approach helps develop a typology which is both indigenous (a classification system which includes categories articulated by the study group) and analytically inducted (where the analyst develops terms to describe categories for which the study group have no labels (Patton, 1990)).

Seven types of supportive functions drawn from the perspectives of residents were identified (Table 7.1). 'Household', 'personal', 'confiding', 'companionship', 'decision making and feedback' were all terms used by residents to describe support received and were deemed appropriate labels for different categories. 'Material' and 'surveillance' were terms devised by the authors which were thought to depict behaviours described by residents. Categorisations were therefore both 'indigenous' as well as analytically devised. Reference is also made to the number of individuals who drew attention to each type of support (Table 7.2).

Table 7.1
Descriptions of seven types of social support

Household	shopping, cooking, cleaning, washing, ironing clothes
Personal	physical help with bathing, dressing, medication, getting up and down stairs
Confiding	confiding relationship, listening
Material	money, gifts, transport
Decision-making and feedback	decision-making, praise, encouragement
Companionship	spending time with someone, talking or sitting silently with person
Surveillance	anticipatory and preventive care 'watching out for'

It is important to remember that social support is a multidimensional concept (Streeter and Franklin, 1992; Florian et al. 1995) and that the categories described are not meant to be mutually exclusive. Though grounded in the accounts of residents themselves, the categories should be regarded purely as an organising guide for the analysis that follows.

Table 7.2
Support Type Distribution

Support type	Mountain View		Greentrees	
	n	%	n	%
Household	8	80	15	100
Personal	5	50	13	87
Confiding	7	70	4	27
Decision-making and feedback	6	60	2	13
Material	7	70	10	67
Companionship	10	100	15	100
Surveillance	0	0	4	27

Household support (N=23)

Household support was referred to as help with daily domestic tasks and included cooking, shopping, cleaning, and washing and ironing clothes. Typical expressions of such support were the following:

Andrew: They [staff] go for the shopping. They give me clean clothes... they make sure I've got them to wear.

Robert: Well they [staff] do everything like. They cook and look after us, so that we are clothed and things like that. They help us with household maintenance you know.

Previous support typologies for people with mental health problems have not featured household support per se (see Carveth and Gottlieb, 1979; Gottlieb, 1983; Rook, 1984; Tardy, 1985). However, it has parallels with instrumental support (Pattison, 1977; Streeter and Franklin, 1992), behavioural assistance (Barrera and Ainley, 1983) which refers to sharing of tasks through physical labour and 'daily and weekly household tasks,' the support types portrayed in the study of elderly people by Qureshi et al. (1989), as well as 'household chores and property maintenance' (Wenger, 1992).

Perceptions of household support - paid chores or social event?

For some residents, particularly those in Greentrees (N=9), cooking and washing were seen as the responsibility of staff since they were viewed as being paid to engage in these tasks.

However, for some individuals support with particular household tasks such as shopping and drawing DSS entitlements had meanings above and beyond 'paid duties'. In general, shopping for some residents in Greentrees (N=6) was talked of as being something they did with staff. Such tasks appeared to have meanings more closely associated with feelings of attachment and friendship, as illustrated in the following comment from Robert:

> They are all my friends in 'Dayspring', all the staff. They help me with living here, house maintenance. I can't confide in them but we go to the post office and we all go shopping together and then we go for a coffee in Siop Nain.

For many residents in Mountain View (N=8) household tasks were often encased within social activities and offered the prospect of reciprocity. Help with shopping and cooking were virtually the only activities linking staff with some residents. This may account for why it was construed by individuals as a form of socialising:

Sarah: My key worker and I, umm, we go shopping and then, umm, go to the café, umm, yes, she comes here for tea or coffee with me and we have a chat.

Household support in this case was therefore a route to conversation but it illustrated that residents and staff sometimes needed an excuse through undertaking chores merely to talk to each other. 'Just sitting talking' to residents did not appear to be on the rehabilitative agenda in Mountain View. Youll and McCourt Perring (1993) found that whereas adequate provision for physical and resource needs was appreciated by people with a range of dependency needs in residential settings, meeting social and emotional needs were valued more highly by residents.

Four residents in Mountain View, (Chris, Sarah, Daniel and Saul) stated that they sometimes went shopping together and would on occasions cook for each other. Sarah provided a good illustration:

> ... I've helped Saul with his shopping because we bought our shopping together with one of the umm, I don't know what you call them... nurses. Oh and also Daniel has made me baked potatoes and what else did we have? We had a coke, a cup of tea, umm not tea, coffee and... anyway I've had quite a few meals with him. I had a meal with him once when we had pancakes and Chris and Gareth came up to my flat on Boxing day last year and I made them a Boxing day dinner. We had chicken for dinner. It was nice too.

Roles and self-worth

For some individuals, involvement in domestic chores was very important as it offered possible routes to the achievement of independence, mastery and self-worth:

Timothy: Well, I see to the greenhouse, tomatoes, cucumber, lettuce and I do the lawns. I do the washing up in the morning as well. These are my jobs. In the afternoon, I go for a walk to the Spar to get things, sometimes I get things for the house. I go on my own. There are people to speak to there.

Richard: I do the garden. I do 'tatoes in the soil and I water the plants and flowers - that's me job.

Walter: I always dry the dishes - are they (Timothy and Sidney) doing them now? Tell [project worker] to call me in when they are going to do them.

These observations from residents would support the findings of Dufåker (1994, p.10) who found that not being able to exert influence over individuals' own situations seemed to influence their quality of life negatively.

However, specific chores assigned to each resident meant that they had a role to play within their own home. Roles within any given social context have long been regarded as significant in developing a sense of self (Mead, 1934), securing identity (Parsons, 1951; Giddens, 1989) and self-worth (McGill, 1987) as well as raising self-esteem (Brown and Harris, 1978; Joseph, 1990; Pilling, 1991). Such characteristics were evident in the cases of Sidney, Walter, Timothy and Frederick who said they washed up and Timothy, Richard and Thomas who proudly stated that they were responsible for gardening for their household. As Thomas himself indicated:

> Well I plant lettuce and busy lizzies but not tomatoes this year. Would you like to see them? (smiling) Would you like to buy a lettuce?

Given that Thomas was inclined to stay silent or at best answer in monosyllables when asked questions, the above comment has added significance in indicating the importance of the activity to his sense of self-esteem. Ascribed social roles therefore have the potential to provide people with esteem (Gottlieb, 1985), helping to boost self-confidence. Ramon (1991) argues that people who leave hospital go through a passage insofar as they are asked to shed one social role and identity for a more socially desirable one. She argues that provision of roles may be a means by which individuals can move towards this desired end.

To this end some individuals repeatedly emphasised their ascribed role as gardener by talking about it in detail. Richard was a case in point:

I mow the lawn and do the potatoes. I always do the potatoes. I mow the lawn for the lady next door as well. I do the digging and cutting. I always do the gardens. Both back and front gardens I do...

Age and physical disability were factors associated with the 'hands on' approach to care generally adopted by staff in Greentrees. However, the oldest and most disabled in terms of general behaviour were also found to be the most able at certain household chores. Qureshi and Walker (1989) argue that dependency is an indicator of the receipt of assistance rather than a need for it (ibid, p.87). In particular, Andrew of 'Hendy' was adept at cleaning and hoovering. Thomas, also of 'Hendy', had expressed his enjoyment with cooking and staff encouraged him to pursue this further. Thomas's specialities were cakes and puddings, particularly rice pudding. His joy of cooking was evident in his smile as he proudly showed people what he had made. He also made sandwiches for his colleagues.

Symbols of independence

Shopping, cooking and gardening had particular importance and value in terms of continued social participation, exchange and reciprocity. To give this up could be an important marker of increased dependency.

Jane, for example, expressed her independence by having the opportunity to clean, shop and cook. Being able to do these chores by herself was symbolic to Jane of this status:

I can look after myself you know. I don't want to go to a nursing home where they do everything for you - no because I can look after myself you see.

Similarly, Sarah and Chris of Mountain View associated the ability to engage in household tasks with independence:

Sarah: Oh yes, I like living in my flat. I'm more independent than in the hospital. I can cook when I want and I look after the place myself.

Chris: I'm independent, you see, Rachel. I buy my own food and then I cook it. I like a fry up best - bacon and eggs.

However, for individuals living in one of the shared flats, failure to tidy and clean it regularly resulted in unkempt conditions (for example cigarette ends and ash littered on the floor). In response, this group was provided with a large proportion of staff time to help clean up. There was evidence that male residents in Mountain View received more support than the two female residents, suggesting a gendered basis to the division of domestic labour.

That others in the same project received domestic support caused a degree of disillusionment among some residents about the aims of community care. This was expressed by those who did not receive similar help or by those who felt that different rules were in operation for different residents. Sarah had a strong view in this connection:

> I think it's terrible - they [staff] said that we had to be independent when we came into the community. That was the whole point of it, that we would do things for ourselves. But the three upstairs in the flat get everything done for them and I don't. I have to do everything myself. I cook and clean and everything whilst the staff do all their washing and everything. Well let them go back up there to hospital if they can't look after themselves...

In summary, there are three key points to be made about household support.

Firstly, this type of support embodied different meanings for individuals. For some it was seen as work for which staff were paid. It was not observed to have any other intrinsic benefits for these individuals. For others help with household tasks was a means of companionship and a route towards friendship.

Secondly, it was also demonstrated that some individuals enjoyed the independence, autonomy, roles and responsibility associated with household chores. With increasing age and disability, such roles were important to individuals, supporting the argument that keeping hold of household tasks can be a valued mark of independence (Wenger, 1992).

Thirdly, some individuals had a particularly keen sense of the 'rules of the game' in relation to receipt of household help and there was some evidence to suggest that these may have been biased against women.

Personal support (N=18)

Personal support included bathing, dressing and medication in the main but also help with mobility as indicated in the following quotes:

Ruth: They [staff] give me a bath... and watch I've got plenty of soap and they buy essential things for me.. help me with personal things.

Chris: My key worker, she helps me to self-medicate by giving me so many tablets per day. Then I get an injection every month.

Personal support may also be found within categories used by others of problem-solving (Gottlieb, 1978), and instrumental (House, 1981) as well as behavioural assistance (Barrera and Ainlay, 1983).

Eight residents from Greentrees and four from Mountain View received support with bathing and dressing. In terms of medication, seventeen residents were undergoing depot injection treatment and were dependent upon staff for at least the provision and regulation of medication, (N=5/10 Mountain View, N=13/15

Greentrees). Personal support, all of it provided by staff, was therefore slightly less prevalent than household care.

Personalised personal support - little things with big meanings

In both projects there were individuals whom staff felt would fail to wash themselves were some kind of support not provided, thus presenting risks to personal hygiene and well-being. Help involved physical tending but was also non routine and individualised.

Help with bathing was construed by some residents (N=6) as having considerable significance for reasons connected to how 'individual attention' was construed. For example, Paul of Mountain View stated that one member of staff 'puts bubble bath in the water and she washes my hair as well. I like that.' Such 'extras' were appreciated and perceived as beyond what staff were usually expected or paid to do. That residents in Mountain View were supposed to engage in self-care with little support from staff may have led to the perception that this kind of care, when provided, was done so voluntarily or out of affection for the individuals concerned.

Such personalised help with bathing and dressing was also the experience of residents in Greentrees (N=8). Ruth, for example, perceived personal care to involve duties carried over from hospital routines, but its meaning for her was highly personalised:

> They've (staff) got a hospital routine you know...They give me a bath and keep me clean and watch if I've plenty of soap and buy me essential things. They give me clean clothes...I like Sheila because she understands me. I can confide in her and she gives me a bath and helps me. She sees that I have enough soap...

This comment illustrates how the meaning of support can be intensified for the recipient by the manner in which people are helped. Support provided in this way can also facilitate the emergence of valued relationships which embodied friendliness, confidentiality and respect. Youll and McCourt Perring (1993) argue that care practices which help to value and appreciate the differences between people are likely to enhance opportunities for people to achieve a sense of fulfilment.

Confiding (N=11)

The accessibility and presence of a confidant, described as someone with whom one can talk about the joys, sorrows and problems of life (Blau, 1973; Wenger, 1984) or in whom one can disclose personal thoughts and feelings or who cares and is there when one needs them (Gottlieb, 1985), has been shown to be a significant predictor of improvement in depressive symptoms (Surtees, 1980; Paykel et al. 1980).

Other studies have highlighted the range of emotionally supportive behaviours that may be provided by a confidant including 'emotionally sustaining behaviour' (Gottlieb, 1978; House, 1981), 'affect' or caring and emotional intimacy (Pattison, 1977; Kahn and Antonucci, 1980) or 'attachment and intimacy' (Weiss, 1974) from which individuals gain a sense of security and place. In this study, confiding behaviours were based on residents' comments about having someone to confide in or to share 'secrets' with. The precondition seemed to be that of a person who could offer a sympathetic, listening ear and in whom one could entrust highly intimate or personal details as indicated below:

Stephen: I can tell [project worker] any worries that I have.

Ruth: I tell [project worker] about my secrets and my worries.

Chris: I can confide in my key worker. It's easy to talk to her.

Only 11/25 residents in this study (N=4 in Greentrees N=7 in Mountain View) named individuals in whom they could confide. Although the proportion of Greentrees residents having confidants was small, the individuals concerned were all project workers. All four residents stated that they received help with bathing and dressing by the same project workers in whom they tended to confide. This illustrates the multi-dimensional character of support. A significant number of residents in Mountain View (7/10) named people in whom they felt they could confide. Confidants included individuals from all network membership categories apart from service contacts.

However only a very small number of residents (N=3/25) felt that they could confide in colleagues from their hospital days. The passage of time and shared experiences were obviously not rites of passage in this regard.

Confiding based on gender and key workers

The majority of people who acted as confidants (N=18) were women (N=14 78%) irrespective of the gender of resident. Female residents had more confidants (mean=3, range=1-5) than their male counterparts (mean=1.2, range=1-2). This supports the findings of studies of other groups which report that women tend to have more intimate and confiding relationships than men (Lowenthal and Haven, 1968; Burke and Weir, 1978; Hirsch, 1979). Traditional sex-role relationships may explain these differences. Women have traditionally been socialised into accepting the nurturing role, a gender construction which manifests itself within segregated conjugal roles as well as divisions of labour in the workforce (see Bott, 1957 and Oakley, 1974).

Staff named as confidants were more often than not key workers, suggesting that the opportunity to become more closely acquainted over time, even when initially prescribed through a formal role relationship, can lead to close and confiding relationships between residents and staff. This was in evidence at both housing projects.

Confiding as a concomitant to friendship

Confiding was found to be the key factor separating 'close' friendship from friendliness. Thus 'best' or 'close' friendship was defined in terms of having opportunities to share intimate thoughts, worries and feelings which are regarded as important for psychological and emotional health (Surtees, 1980; Leavy, 1983) and morale (Wenger et al. 1991). This point is exemplified in the following quotes:

Stephen: Dorothy [project worker] is my friend. I have conversations with her. I could tell my worries to her. I like her the best.

Matthew: Don [staff] is very important to me. He is one of my best friends. I'd miss Don if he wasn't here. He is my closest friend. I can confide in him...

Saul: Chris [resident] is my friend. I can talk about lots of things with Chris you know, confide in him what I would like to do and I discuss things with him. I tell him what my plans are and he tells me what he wants from here. He told me that he wanted to move out of here but he's not prepared to break the rules you see.

Confiding and personal support

It was observed that residents tended to receive help with bathing and dressing from the same project workers with whom they could confide. Although it is argued that expressive aspects of caring do not have to come wrapped around practical tasks (Qureshi and Walker, 1989, p.23), the evidence here indicates that residents preferred designated members of staff to help them with personal care tasks, suggesting that there were additional intrinsic benefits to individuals. Particularly evident were factors connected to the fulfilment of affective needs and the maintenance of a positive self-image, for example the ability to express private thoughts knowing that confidences would be respected, being valued as a person, being able to enter freely into exchanges of expressive behaviour and so on.

In this case personal care took place in a context where intimacy was the key ingredient together with time, and having someone to listen and take interest in the person, and it was this that appeared to facilitate the emergence of valued relationships. This lends some support to the findings of Weiss (1974) who argues that 'attachment and intimacy' are provided in relationships from which individuals gain a sense of security and place. Feelings can be expressed freely and without self-consciousness, and in such relationships individuals feel comfortable and at home.

Confiding deficits

Finally, as stated earlier, a significant number of residents (N=14) could not confide in anyone.

The absence of emotional support is interesting in the light of previous research regarding the primary importance of a confiding relationship (Caplan, 1974; Gottlieb, 1978; House, 1981; Cohen and Wills, 1985). Nevertheless, out of those who had no confidants, none stated, when asked, that they would like someone to confide in. It appears therefore that for individuals who have existed for so long without it, confiding as a form of support may no longer be regarded as having a central significance to their lives.

Decision-making and feedback (N=8)

Eight individuals in the study considered that they received support in the form of decision-making and feedback which might be positive (encouragement, praise) or negative (disapproval). Six residents in Mountain View stated that they received this kind of support compared with only two at Greentrees.

The category of decision-making and feedback bears a resemblance to what Barrera and Ainlay (1983) described as guidance (meaning offering advice, information or instruction) and feedback (meaning the provision of feedback about their behaviours, thoughts or feelings). In almost every case, decision-making and feedback was provided by paid staff. Only Saul reported that he received guidance from a fellow resident:

> I can talk about lots of things with Chris you know, confide in him what I would like to do and I discuss things with him. I tell him what my plans are...

The salience of encouragement - key to self-esteem

In the present study the experience of encouragement was highly salient for those who received it (N=4) and was central to understanding their self-esteem. Jane provided a good example:

> They all [staff] tell me I'm doing very well you know. I can look after myself you know. Roy, the manager told me that I was doing very well for my age... I can look after myself you see... even though I'm old, I can cook for myself...

This comment also shows that positive feedback about everyday functioning was a marker of independence for Jane. Similarly, Daniel stated that his key worker encouraged him to stick with his diet and Chris said that staff encouraged him to budget his finances, praising him when he had managed to save money. Positive feedback regarding how residents were 'getting on' in their community locations was appreciated by other residents in Mountain View, as indicated by Gareth:

> I do these things...washing and I have a shave. If I let myself go down, they don't like me but give me thanks if I try...

The importance of decision-making

People with psychiatric problems tend to have difficulties with making decisions (House, 1981). Residents reported a need for support with decisions which were important for their day-to-day functioning. For three individuals in Mountain View, this applied mostly to finances and medication. Sarah stated that her key worker and social workers helped her to fill in forms for attendance allowance and Daniel stated that whilst he wanted 'to go off me tablets because they don't do me any good', he intended to talk this over with his key worker before making a final decision. Albert also argued that it was his key worker who helped him make decisions about whether to ring his relatives or not.

The contradiction of decision-making

Staff at Mountain View were reluctant to intervene in people's lives and this sometimes led to difficulties when certain residents decided not to wash or dress properly, illustrating a tension between philosophy and individual needs. In the case of Saul, his decision to 'do as I want' led to him being labelled by project workers as 'difficult and unpopular'. He was eventually advised by staff to return to hospital because, in the words of the deputy manager, 'the Mountain View regime (of self-help) was not suitable for him'.

By contrast, in Greentrees only James and Ruth reported that they had help with decision-making, in both cases in connection with choosing what clothes to wear or buy. This contradicted the reports of staff who stated that a large part of their role consisted of making decisions for residents. Observations confirmed this. However, decision-making by staff for individuals was not always deemed appropriate or appreciated by residents. For example, staff decided that James should only be allowed a certain amount of money at a time since to prevent him from spending too much on sweets. James felt that this was an infringement of his freedom:

James: I don't get any money here at all. The pension which I sign for they put that in the bank. But I'd rather have the money to put in the Post Office you know.

R: Have you asked them then if you can do that?

James: Eh.. no. I haven't no, because they come to me to sign the pension books and put the money in the bank. That's all there is to it. I didn't have any say in it you know. I'd like more so that I can buy things.

Support provided is therefore not necessarily support needed or required, supporting the idea that misguided help can have unintended negative effects (Ell, 1996).

Material support (N=17)

This category referred to support in the form of money and material exchanges. Whilst transport was difficult to place within the typology, it was subsumed here since economic exchange was involved and it did not fit easily into the other support categories.

It was found that use of public transport by residents was minimal. In Mountain View only Peter and Daniel used the local bus service. Staff with cars would often provide lifts. For more organised trips a hospital mini-bus was used for transport. Similarly a significant number of residents (N=10/15) in Greentrees expressed a preference to be taken by staff on excursions in cars rather than travel independently by using public transport:

Ruth: She [project worker] takes me to chapel in the car. I like to go out in the car.

Cigarettes were also included as a material item in this type of support as residents felt that they were a drain on their own resources and so the giving and receiving of cigarettes was significant as a form of material exchange:

Sidney: We [residents] always give each other cigs.

Financial assistance was received mainly from family members. The literature on the social networks of general population samples suggests that even though kin may be separated by distance, financial aid can still be a predominant helping behaviour (Rosser and Harris, 1965). In the present study only three residents reported financial assistance from kin. Limited financial help for individuals may well be due to the fact that contact for most residents is restricted to 'extended' kin whose sense of obligation to individuals cannot be expected to be as great as that of close family members.

Other types of material aid came from different sources. Transport for the majority of residents (N=24/25) was provided by staff or service contacts. In only once case, Robert, was transport provided through the informal support network. He received a lift to and from choir practice from a social acquaintance:

Robert: I get a lift back from choir practice sometimes like.. I get a lift back with one of the choir members. Oh yes, they are pretty good like that.

On the other hand, the exchange of money, cigarettes, cups of tea and other gifts provided by either relatives or other residents was mediated almost entirely through informal networks. Quite a large number of residents (N=17) in both projects received material support from family members and staff in the form of money, gifts and transport. However, it was difficult to discern the significance of these for residents.

Whilst cars were rented for residents in Greentrees all three residents in each house tended to be driven around at the same time. The experience was therefore little changed from the days of hospital mini-buses. In Mountain View, hospital practices were repeated with the few organised excursions involving a hospital mini-bus. Whilst residents were encouraged to use public transport, they became accustomed to being taken everywhere by staff.

The salience of cigarettes

The exchange of cigarettes was perhaps the most significant form of material support to residents and the type most often spoken about. Since, for many residents, smoking was a central component of their lives the receiving of cigarettes became very important to them. In effect, the exchange of these commodities became a way in which residents could help each other. It provided the basis of affinity between them and with staff. It was also observed that residents would often automatically light a cigarette for staff members as well as for themselves. In fact the statement 'cigarette?' was often a form of greeting. Similarly, the buying of tea for one another was an important means of exchange between individuals, especially for those living in Mountain View. Jane in particular valued such provision:

Jane: ...well, you know my friend Carl (hospital contact), well he buys me a cup of tea sometimes. Yes, he buys me a pot of tea in Kwiks. I like it when someone buys me a cup of tea.

Such behaviour was reminiscent of that observed in the hospital coffee bar during the pilot study. Dunn et al. (1990) have reported that 'the purchase and exchange of commodities, such as tea and cigarettes, appear to serve a social function for this long-stay population equivalent to that in conversations of healthy people'. From the present evidence the same could be said of those now living in community settings.

Companionship (N=25)

Willmott (1987) argues that the opportunity to spend time with someone is the first stage within processes that may lead to friendship. In this study, companionship manifested itself in two ways. The first was in the form of everyday conversation between two or more people:

Robert: Well when we (other residents and hospital contacts) are in the [day centre] we chat and talk. And the warden of the church, well he's a very good friend of mine. Oh I talk to him every Sunday and on a Friday night when I go to choir practice like.

Gareth: I talk to the other residents and they talk to me. They are part of my life.

Interpersonal dialogue has previously been acknowledged as an essential aspect of social interaction (Buber, 1965) which Dufåker (1994, p.7) posits as an 'existential prerequisite for human life'. The second was simply sharing time with someone which did not necessarily involve verbal interaction:

Andrew: I don't talk to Stephen and Thomas, not much, but we go to the pub for a pint.

Whilst there were overlaps between companionship and confiding, residents made a distinction between talking about everyday matters and sharing intimate thoughts and ideas. Table 7.2 shows that all 25 residents reported companionship as a form of support. As with material aid, companionship was found to include both formal sources (mostly staff) and informal sources (mostly residents and social acquaintances).

Companionship appeared to be the main value that all individuals attributed to their relationships with others. Companionship was either conversational or involved just having someone to sit with.

Conversational companionship

Whilst residents referred to 'close friends' as people they could confide in, 'friendship' was linked to 'talking about everyday matters'. However a distinction was drawn between members of staff who conversed with them and those who did not:

Ruth: Sheila and Patrick (staff) are my friends because they talk to me. Patrick has a little girl now and she's a year old and has little teeth. Patrick said to me I know you like little girls and you will be kind to them and so he brings his little girl to see me. Yes he's very good, he always talks to me even though I know he has to do his work and can't spend all day with me. But the other one [project worker], he's no good. I don't respect him.

In such cases conversation and the time taken to converse came to be regarded as an important indicator of friendship.

If they wanted, individuals could spend time entertaining guests in their own rooms or elsewhere though it was an option not commonly pursued. It was more usual for residents to sit in the communal lounge. This was not necessarily a positive preference but more a reaction to the fact that no structured activities were available. Residents like Sarah offered the view that the communal lounge gave her a 'break from my flat and I can chat to people and watch television'. Conversations tended to centre around cigarettes, teasing or reminiscing about the 'old days' in hospital. Hence fellow residents provided an important source of company.

Silent companionship

Apart from conversation, companionship could also involve passive behaviour such as just 'sitting' next to other residents. It was not uncommon to see individuals seated together but saying very little to one another. This type of behaviour perhaps indicates that shades of institutionalism are still apparent despite new community settings. It was akin to patterns of behaviour reported by Dunn et al. (1990) who categorised residents' friends as 'patients who have a well defined group of companions with whom they spend their time, sitting, chatting and drinking tea, although often with long periods in silence'.

Companionship deficits

Nevertheless, there was no doubt that residents wanted more company and, in particular, people to talk to. Jane, Albert and Peter all stated that they would like to 'meet more people'. Jane also mentioned that whilst she was friendly with Sarah, she would have liked another female friend in Mountain View. This was because Sarah was prone to mood swings which Jane found difficult to handle, stating 'sometimes she doesn't talk to me or will look at me - she's funny like that'.

Sunday was a particularly difficult day for individuals. In David's words there was 'nothing to do and no one to see'. For Jane, Sunday was also a reflective time in which she missed her relatives. Lehr (1981) suggests that extra-familial social life is a protection against loneliness in old age. However, 'protection' of this kind was an unlikely situation since many residents had either lost touch with or had no relatives. These points are illustrated by Jane:

Jane: I don't like Sunday, no I don't. It's too quiet. There are not as many people around as on the weekdays. I think of my brother and my mother and my father. I've got no one... I feel very lonely.

The quote above is indicative of expressed feelings of eleven residents though only three were from Greentrees. Although crude, such responses were also similar to those found by Wenger (1984). She also found that the very lonely were twice as likely to have small support networks. However, in the present study a high percentage (73%, N=8) of those who expressed loneliness and a need for companions were residents at Mountain View. They had larger social networks than those in Greentrees (mean = 34.1 and 19.5 respectively). Each individual at Mountain View lived within close proximity to nine other residents. In these regards loneliness did not appear to be associated with small social networks or social isolation. This finding supports findings from studies of older people which have shown that there is no direct relationship between social isolation and loneliness (Hadley and Webb, 1974; Lebowitz, 1980), and that even those living with others may be lonely (Wenger, 1984).

Other factors would therefore have to account for feelings of loneliness. From the evidence provided above, it seems more likely that conversation was the most valued form of companionship. It was this rather than just 'having someone there' that individuals in Mountain View linked to alleviating loneliness. Albert stated that he would have liked more people to visit and converse with him. However, since he perceived the other residents as 'ill' he felt that he had little in common with them and so never sought their company.

The key to this dilemma appears to be that some residents did not, or felt that they could not, communicate with their fellow residents in conversations that went beyond everyday occurrences such as bartering for cigarettes. This is poignantly illustrated by Peter:

> I'm lonely, really lonely... I don't know no-one... but I can't get on with them up there (Mountain View). I can't talk to them - they're all high on drugs...

The three residents (Sidney, Ruth and Matthew) in Greentrees who expressed a desire to meet new people were observed to be particularly talkative individuals compared to others such as Owain and Thomas who were very quiet.

In Chapter 3, ratings scales for psychiatric state (KRS) and behaviour (REHAB) revealed that residents in Greentrees generally had greater incoherence and poverty of speech as well as speech disturbance than their Mountain View counterparts. This may have accounted for limited communication. On the other hand, project workers suggested that during hospital days conversation between residents and others had always been limited, as if reflecting institutionalised silence. Thus, for some residents, meeting new people to talk to was not necessarily an important expressed need. This was illustrated by Stephen from 'Hendy':

> I don't want anyone to talk to. I'm happy as I am. I like to just sit here on the comfy chair and watch television with the other two [residents].

In summary, whilst communication may have been generally more important for individuals in Mountain View, companionship was perceived as a valued support by all residents. Nevertheless, the company provided was not necessarily the kind that was needed or preferred.

Surveillance (N=4)

Despite its rather covert character, surveillance was referred to by a small number of residents. They described it in terms of keeping a watchful eye out for one another and there were occasions when it led to more direct intervention such as enlisting further support from staff when someone got into personal difficulty. It must be remembered that residents knew each other's ways extremely well and they could be very attentive to each other's needs. For example:

Robert: Well, I feel for Howard. He's quite poorly - it's hard for him. The staff, they never saw him like I did in hospital. He gets so he doesn't know what he's doing. I watch out for him like - oh yes.

There was an awareness that staff acted in this way though only a few residents, all at Greentrees, referred explicitly to it.

Preventive care or 'monitoring at a distance' was observed in all the Greentrees houses as well as Mountain View. However, whilst 'preventive' often led to 'supervisory' and/or 'instrumental' care by staff in Greentrees, staff generally stopped short of anything more than 'preventive' care in Mountain View, reflecting the adopted laissez-faire model of care. This meant that people like Saul and Gareth were allowed to deteriorate in their physical appearance, personal hygiene and general well-being as a matter of their 'own choice'.

Only four residents, all from Greentrees, had an awareness that they were being 'watched' by staff and colleagues. Matthew of 'Brangwyn' stated that his fellow resident, Edward, 'watched out' for him. This was confirmed by Edward himself.

On the other hand, none of the residents in Mountain View mentioned surveillance at all. Surveillance was not on the Mountain View staff agenda as it implied invasion of privacy. Only Albert was surreptitiously 'monitored at a distance' by staff due to his having grand mal seizures, a symptom of his epilepsy. However, whilst staff tried hard to preserve each resident's freedom and privacy by not engaging in surveillance, it appeared that this was construed by residents as disinterestedness. This was noted by Gareth:

> the staff don't bother us here, they don't look after us like, they don't take much notice see...they just leave us to get on with it...

Discussion

This chapter has attempted to disaggregate the idea of support into different categories. Six of the support categories have been identified in previous studies of elderly people living in the community (Qureshi et al. 1989; Wenger, 1992) as well as reports of clinical populations (Pinneau, 1975; Caplan, 1976). However, the added category of 'surveillance' identified in this study would tend to validate the inclusion of 'invisible care' in Bowers' (1987) typology.

An indication of the deficiencies in support experienced by individuals has also been given. Not all residents were found to be in receipt of all seven types of support. Eight residents (32%) indicated that they received three or less types of support, suggesting marked individual differences. Residents in Mountain View generally were in receipt of slightly more support types (mean=5) than those in Greentrees (mean=4). There was a significant positive link between social network size and support variety ($r=0.4$ $p<.05$) suggesting that people with larger networks are more likely to be able to draw upon a greater variety of support.

The distribution of support types also varied between projects. As shown in Table 7.2, support for residents in Greentrees was concentrated more on personal and household tasks, these being provided mainly by project workers. Again this can be explained by the different care practices adopted in both projects. In Mountain View, the supply of support from staff was hindered by the apparent contradiction between individual needs and laissez-faire philosophy.

Nevertheless, the most striking finding of the study was the lack of confiding and conversational companionship. In particular, residents in Mountain View wished for more relationships with others having shared interests and with people in whom they could share their intimate thoughts and ideas.

Summary

- The findings reaffirm the multi-dimensional character of support.
- Apparently mundane forms of support from staff and others can have a particular significance to residents in how they look upon their independence and self-image. Ascribed social roles were important in this connection.
- Contexts where privacy was required, as for example in the case of bathing, offered the potential for intimate and confiding relationships to grow between residents and staff.
- Key worker arrangements appeared to help confiding relationships to develop.
- A high proportion of residents did not report confiding relationships.
- Loneliness and support network size appeared to be unrelated.
- Feedback and encouragement from staff was a key to understanding self-image. These qualities were less in evidence where a laissez-faire system was present.

- Reciprocity between residents was mediated in the main by the exchange of cigarettes.
- Although most residents valued companionship, some wishing for more, others did not wish to associate with their peers as this was equated with the perpetuation of an illness label.
- Lack of planned activities and day opportunities reduced the number of contexts in which new relationships could be formed.

8 Residents' views of their relationships with different supporters

> Perceived social support is not an isolated perception that comes into play only when individuals are confronted by a stressful situation that demands coping behaviour. It is part of a constellation of cognitions that derive from a history of social interactions and accounts for differences in interpretations of situations, the motives of others, and beliefs about what others are 'really like'.
>
> (Sarason et al. 1994, p.109)

Users' views of community care have commonly been based on questionnaires such as the Patient Attitude Questionnaire, (Thornicroft et al. 1993) which rate attitudes and satisfaction levels (see Pickard, 1992; Holloway and Faulkner, 1994; Brabbins et al. 1995). Similarly, attitudes towards staff have often been limited to highly structured forms of questioning (Perkins et al. 1992; Dayson, 1992; Holloway and Faulkner, 1994; Reda, 1994). In this chapter case study material is analysed to assess how individuals construe their attachments to others. Since the findings about support network structure revealed five principal membership categories, these are used here as convenient headings to review what further dimensions about the social lives of individuals could be added by analysis of the qualitative data.

Resident-staff relationships - formal or informal?

Resident-staff dichotomy - transfer of the medical model?

Most residents in Greentrees perceived project workers as nursing staff who were there to help run the house, suggesting that the relationship was functional but formal for them. This was illustrated by the language used by residents about project workers. Only 6/15 referred to staff by name, whilst 9/15 residents referred impersonally to project workers, suggesting an element of social distancing:

Richard: They listen to the television and chat amongst themselves... they give me cigarettes.

Ruth: They've got to do their work. They go and do their work, they can't stay long with me.... the nurses told me I had a secret and they gave me a secret because I'd been good.

Robert: Oh the staff don't sit with us when we eat - they make it you see.

One of the factors underlying the social distance felt between residents and staff was personal history. With individuals having been hospitalised for many years it was difficult for them to shed images of staff as nurses. However, this social distancing was also found to be based on residents' compliance with house and rehabilitative requirements worked out in both projects. Failure to do so resulted in chastisement or in the labelling of individuals as unpopular.

For example, Saul was a particularly unpopular resident at Mountain View because in the eyes of staff he did not comply with the ground rules about 'self help'. Although able to engage in domestic tasks, he exercised his 'right to choose' not to comply with the rehabilitation aims in his care plan. A chain smoker, he coughed continuously and spat onto the floor. Staff responded negatively to this and he was eventually readmitted to hospital. One member of staff at Mountain View summed it up thus:

> It was a difficult decision, but it was hard with someone that wasn't popular. None of the staff liked him and he didn't get on with the other residents. We tried everything but he didn't respond. This place couldn't offer him the type of care he needed.

This illustration suggests that some things have changed little from the 'model patient' described in the literature (Goffman, 1961; Denzin, 1968). Smith and Thrasher (1968), in their study of patient roles within psychiatric hospitals, found that a refusal by patients to conform to norms within the hospital, such as keeping appointments with therapists, evoked the strongest negative sanctions.

Although Saul was observed to be the most unpopular resident within Mountain View, other residents moved in and out of popularity depending on how their behaviour and role performance was observed. Occasionally some residents decided to stop cooking their own meals, which led to accusations about individuals 'playing the sick role'. However, there was a connection with key worker relationships here.

Informal and formal key workers

In Mountain View, key workers were generally seen as the most important staff members to individuals. Although individuals were free to ask anyone for help they tended to feel that they could only approach their key workers with personal questions or worries. An example of this heavy reliance upon one particular member of staff was Sarah. She preferred to wait until her key worker was on duty rather than approach someone else:

> It's important to get along with the staff but it varies, depends on the staff. You see, I'm in contact more with my key worker and my social worker than what I am with anybody else. I get on with them all but I do more with my key worker because she is my key worker...

Although a formal key worker system did not exist in Greentrees, in some houses an informal key worker system was in evidence where members of staff had developed routines about taking particular residents to particular activities. This was also observed in Mountain View where some members of staff gravitated towards particular residents even if they were not their 'key clients'. Again 'popular' residents were those who were willing to comply with house policy. Likewise, residents also had 'favourite' members of staff whom they 'did a lot with'. Thus there was a tendency for some staff and residents to gravitate towards each other.

Quasi-family relationships?

It was suggested in Chapter 5 that the provision of a homely environment had been positively encouraged by local policy statements and management. Variants of the family model had been adopted by staff within each of the Greentrees households to the extent that staff perceived the residential environment to replicate family roles and functions. Similarly, Dufåker (1994) found that the longer the study group were ill, the more likely that professionals became a substitute for socially attributed as well as voluntary contacts.

Ruth was able to draw comparisons with other relatives, living and dead:

> I don't wish to stay here too long. I've got relatives to go to. I'd like to go to my home town. I could go to my relations' house too. It used to be my grandmother's house. I mustn't forget about them. They were important people.

Similarly, Jane equated the relationship she had with some project workers with that of a kinship tie. She regarded the individual who helped her physically as her 'daughter', stating: 'I've taken her as my daughter'. Jane also looked upon herself as 'an old woman' in the aged maternal role in which children look after their aged parents. Staff with whom she had a close relationship thus came to be regarded as substitute children. Jane's perceptions of staff as quasi-relatives may have been a symptom of her longing for kinship relationships which had previously been severed during her hospitalisation.

Staff did not wear uniforms and were regarded by residents as 'project workers' to 'help' them rather than nurse them. As described earlier they were recruited from a range of occupational groups and brought a variety of professional or non-professional work experiences to their present work roles. This was another factor serving to blur the distinction between the helpers and the helped. In another context Bulmer (1986) has argued that the short training and low status of homecare workers can be associated with reduced social distance between clients and themselves, this being a potentially important factor in creating trust between relative strangers.

Resident-family relationships

As explained earlier, most of the study group had never married, there were few family contacts, and contact with family members was very much a function of length of hospitalisation, supporting the findings of Holmes-Eber and Riger (1990).

Perceptions of lost family contact

Two distinctive value positions were struck concerning the absence of kin. Five residents desperately wanted contact with family members. Absence of such contact was construed by them to mean that kin had forgotten them or did not think of them. This was exemplified by Jane who wished to see more of her niece and nephew:

> I've only got my niece and nephew. My nephew never contacts me. He never writes. My niece writes to me. I'd like to see her more often.

On the other hand, five residents did not especially want contact. The main reason for this appeared to be that relationships with kin had broken down at some point through the course of the illness and consequent upon the individual's admission to hospital. An observation by Peter illustrates the reluctance some residents felt about renewing contact with family:

> I've got four brothers... eh, they know where I am, you know, I'm not pushing it to see 'em you know... it's not important to keep in touch with them. I don't want them coming down and seeing me here... because it's degrading. I think so anyway... a place like this, I don't have to be in a place like this.

Peter's comment also gives some clues as to why contact with family members is not always pursued. Some residents retain an acute sense of stigma about being hospitalised, even associating 'ordinary housing' with hospitalisation, so maintaining a hesitancy about maintaining active social ties with family and relatives. Others such as Sarah and Gareth felt that some family members had moved on in their lives and that contact would be inconvenient and disruptive to them:

Gareth: I would see my sister but I don't like to bother her. She has a family and little children and I don't want to interfere.

For others, such as Walter and James, it was more a case of having learned with the passage of time to cope with the absence of kin.

Nevertheless Wellman (1981) also argues that where immediate kin are absent, extended kin can become more important to individuals. Such replacement of network members has been noted before (Wenger, 1984). Similarly Shanas (1979) refers to the 'principle of substitution' in this connection. This system of network member substitution was found to be in operation with some residents who perceived relationships with available kin to be very important to them with serial order tending to take the form of siblings first (Gareth, Sarah, Paul, Daniel, Chris, Robert, Richard, Timothy, Sidney and Edward), then aunts (Albert), and cousins or other extended kin (Jane).

Importance of family contact

For the 15 residents who maintained contact with their families, three means of contact were in evidence: visits, letters and telephone calls.

In Mountain View 4/9 residents received family visits whereas 5/9 had to take the initiative and visit their kin. In Greentrees, 6/15 individuals received visits from their relatives. Visiting had increased since residents' resettlement, staff stating that some relatives were more prepared to visit individuals now that they were out of hospital. As stated by one member of staff, 'they (siblings) wouldn't visit him in hospital but they do now'. The stated reasons for this were to do with the community environment in which residents now lived which ostensibly was free of the hospital stigma, though, as reported earlier, this was a perception not necessarily shared by residents.

Nevertheless, most residents had to take the initiative if they wanted face-to-face contact with kin. Those who valued family contact were often not content with this. This was particularly true of Jane and Albert, with Albert desperately wanting to visit his aunt and uncle:

> I wanted to visit them but my uncle said it wouldn't be right enough or something like that for me to come down, despite my having paid them to go on the buses after they came once. Then my key worker said she would take me down in the car and she spoke to my aunt and uncle about it, but they still said it wouldn't be that easy for me to get out and see them.

This illustration is supported by related research (Barry et al. 1990) which found that a high percentage of residents going through the resettlement process, 31 per cent, were dissatisfied with family contact. Although relatives of individuals in the study were more likely to phone and write letters than visit, this was restricted to Christmas and birthdays with residents on the whole taking the initiative in these specific regards. Only two residents had 'phone calls from family members once a week or more often. Residents reported that such letters and phone calls were important to them as they conveyed the sense that someone 'cared for them'. For the individuals concerned this adds confirmation to the view that contact by phone and letter can enable relationships to be active and intimate over long distances (Bell, 1968; Wenger, 1992). Furthermore, the telephone is an important channel through which emotional support in the form of confiding can take place, Sarah using this means to confide in her sister and ex-husband.

Links between residents and kin members were therefore rather tenuous, and for the vast majority these no longer had significance for them apart from a few who desperately wanted contact. This contrasts sharply with studies of the elderly (Wenger, 1992) and frail elderly people at home (Qureshi et al. 1989; Qureshi and Walker, 1989) where family members are of particular significance in people's lives.

However, since these individuals tended to name more staff in their networks as providers of support it is likely that, in the absence of family members, others had become more important. This was posited by Johnson (1983) who found in a study of post-hospitalised elderly individuals that persons outside the family were more likely to be called upon to help non-married patients than those who were married.

Ties with other residents

Common history - common bond or hindrance?

As explained in Chapter 6, experiences of hospital life had taken up a very large part of individuals' lives and it appeared that this common bond was responsible for holding them together as a group of companions. This is illustrated by Sarah:

> Sometimes in the evening I go to the pub for about an hour with Chris. And sometimes I go to the café with Gareth. Chris will come to me and I'll say 'oh I'm fed up tonight' and I'll ask Chris to go to the pub with me or he'll ask me. He's asked me to go tonight actually. I've known him since 1975. We took shock treatment together. He remembers me there and I remember him. Oh yes and Gareth and, umm, Albert and Paul and David of course I knew on the ward but of course now I'm more friendly with them. I, umm, speak a lot to David a lot more now than what I did on the ward. We were friendly but I only saw them going up and down the corridors or in the shop or in the coffee bar or in the disco, umm, outside in the grounds or if they came to the ward for a cup of tea

with other friends. We used to do that a lot you know, move from ward to ward, have cups of tea from people and then they'd introduce you to somebody and you'd get to know a lot in hospital like that. David's made friends with other people but he will introduce me in the café if I'm on my own or if I'm with friends of mine or friends from here. No David is a good lad.

Sarah's quote was confirmed by Chris in a later conversation:

Chris: Umm, some nights I go the pub with Sarah. She drinks orange squash and I drink vodka and orange.

However, when the fieldworker talked to individuals away from the group, it would often emerge that they did not wish to be associated with 'ex-psychiatric patients'. For example:

David: ...a lot of people in Mountain View I can't communicate with you know, they're in a world of their own, they're on medication, they're on drugs, they're out of their heads you know...

Walter: I don't want to go to no day centre 'cos they are all nuts there.

Peter: I don't have anything to do with the other residents. All they are interested in is fags.

Gareth: I don't want anyone up here from the hospital 'cos they are all institutionalised.

This statement by Gareth was interesting in light of the fact that he still ventured up to the hospital:

I go up to there (hospital) and I talk with Nick. He's a pal to me, little Nick. He's mental you know, he's mental. There is something the matter with him. Aye, I talk to a few there. There's Tommy, he's epileptic, a patient with the doctor. And Roderick, I've known him since he was a pretty young man. And Nick, he's about 70 years old now and he had a leucotomy on his brain. I was in the ward with them. They are part of my life.

These observations from David, Gareth, Walter and Peter seem to suggest that certain individuals can harbour feelings of ambiguity towards others with mental illness. On the one hand, such relationships offer solidarity in a common predicament but on the other hand they may call into question the potential for their participation within the wider community (Barham and Hayward, 1991, p.55). Such individuals still appear to feel a sense of stigma by association with other (mentally ill) residents. In this sense the group living arrangement can constrain their opportunities to develop new relationships with 'ordinary' people. For example, it was very rare for individuals to bring any friends or acquaintances back to their homes. Nevertheless, with other hospital residents being the only people to share the same experiences it is understandable that these relationships are not easily severed.

Leadership, status and power

The discussion so far has shown that residents in this study form a social group constituted by characteristics linked to their shared experiences of hospitalisation. Social groups are defined as a set of individuals who identify with each other, provide moral support from doing so, whilst sustaining a sense of hostility to outgroups (Giddens, 1992). Such groups also possess organisational properties including division of labour and leadership roles to which status and power are linked. The advantages of leadership for individual awareness and self-esteem have been well documented (Weber, 1958; Smelser, 1963 and Pilling, 1991) and the adoption of individual household 'roles' described earlier found to mediate residents' sense of self-worth.

However, individuals can only reach positions of leadership and become effective in what they do if favourable social conditions exist (Giddens, 1992). In the case of residents in this study, there was little opportunity for residents to assume leadership roles in their own home environment. Elsewhere Morris (1993) has described how, in the case of people with disabilities, dependency and lack of individual control over individuals' own lives can lead to a sense of powerlessness and frustration.

One of the few means by which residents could express leadership, status and power was through the giving and selling of cigarettes. This was demonstrated by the following extract from field notes made one evening at Mountain View:

> Sarah and Saul leave the lounge. David, Gareth and Paul remain. Paul begins to beg for a cigarette from David.
>
> Paul: Cigarette David?
>
> David: They all come to me for cigs Rachel.
>
> David smiles and starts to roll a cigarette for Paul. Gareth then stands by David, and David after some period of time offers him a cigarette. Gareth then turns on Paul saying he's a scrounger.
>
> David: Now now Gareth, you wouldn't hit Paul would you or do anything to him would you?

This observation illustrates how residents can get into exploitative relationships with one-another, using cigarettes as the vehicle to maintain status positions. This was similar to the findings of Nelson et al. (1992) who argued that the provision of unsupportive transactions within reciprocal relationships in which one individual was able to exhibit assertiveness was related to mastery or perceived control of that individual's life.

Interestingly, whilst residents in Mountain View moved in and out of 'buying' dominance through cigarettes, Saul had status above and beyond this. This was linked to his refusal to comply with house rules, his insistence on 'his own way' and the use of threatening behaviour in order to get what he wanted. That he was so unpopular with the staff at Mountain View heightened his status with some residents. Saul's use of pressure to be supplied with cigarettes is shown below:

> Daniel [sitting by fieldworker on the minibus] began to talk asking her what she did last night. He lit a cigarette. Saul's face came between them and he asked:
>
> Saul: Can I have a cig Dan?
>
> Daniel: No.
>
> Saul: Just one. I'll give you one back when we get there.
>
> Daniel: No.
>
> Saul: Just one.
>
> Daniel then proceeded to roll a cigarette and gave it to Saul.
>
> Saul: Ta Dan.

Saul's unpopularity with staff and 'bad' behaviour was admired by some residents and he exploited this to maintain authority over fellow residents. This pattern of behaviour was exaggerated by the fact that cigarettes were one of the few items that individuals could offer one another. In the absence of developed relationships, the exchange of cigarettes thus became very significant. It formed or made a statement about how or what the relationship was.

However, at Greentrees, the 'giving up' of smoking was regarded as a social progression as well as a healthy option. Therefore, as a matter of care practice the supply of matches was restricted. Consequently, in some houses, residents would continually walk around with a cigarette in their hand asking for a light. However, the same form of surreptitious exchange between residents was observed out of sight of the staff.

For other residents, friendships emerged out of companionship:

Chris: Jane is a bit like me mother but I feel like I've known Sarah all my life. Saul and I have entertainment together. We make coffee for each other, give each other fags, make sure that we're alright and look after each other socially. We make chat and conversation. Sarah, well she's very unpredictable you know. She's terrible, like Jekyll and Hyde, but she makes me things like bacon and bread and butter sandwiches and, umm, waffles and deep fried chips.

Feelings about the friendship, albeit at times ambivalent, between Chris and Sarah was reciprocated by Sarah soon after Chris died:

Sarah: I knew Chris very well. He was a good friend. Oh he was lovely. He used to tell me he loved me. He used to come up for coffee and he'd put his arm around me and he'd never fail to tell me he loved me. He bought me a little duck to put in my bathroom. Time heals but how long... how long?

For Greentrees residents friendship was reserved principally for fellow house mates and project workers rather than colleagues in other project houses:

Andrew: They are all my friends at 'Hendy' - Stephen and Thomas and all the staff.

Robert: We go to the others' houses but only Richard and Howard are close to me 'cos they live with me.

Environmental influences on relationships between residents

The absence of reported friendships across houses within Greentrees was somewhat different from that found by Meltzer et al. (1994). In a study of three group homes for ex-psychiatric patients, Meltzer and colleagues found that relationships became more cohesive, with an increase in the number of network connections between residents one year after discharge. More significantly, the strongest relationships among residents frequently crossed household boundaries.

That the selection procedure for resident allocation to houses in the present study had been very carefully managed could explain the relative cohesiveness of relationships within as opposed to between houses. Management had sought to place individuals together on the basis of the expressed choices of individuals and by staff observation regarding who were 'known friends'. Abrahamson et al. (1989) have advocated the significance of a period of preparation in sustaining and reviving old social networks before leaving hospital. Furthermore, Dayson (1992), using evidence from a study of two group homes, emphasises the value of the formation of patients into cohesive groups before discharge as a means of enhancing the chances of producing successful households in the community.

In a study of social networks in two group homes, Dayson (1992) found that in one, where patients with a range of ability were put together, residents were found to be cohesive, but in another, in which this type of social mix did not exist, individuals were relatively disconnected. Dayson argued that what began as a socially mixed group was more likely to lead to a mutually supportive hierarchy. Chahal and Lee-Jones (1993) in a five year follow up of the same group investigated by Dayson showed that the cohesiveness of the hierarchical relationship in the first home had developed, and more relationships had come into existence. In contrast, although a core group in the second home had developed both confiding and reciprocal relationships, the social bonds outside this group remained haphazard and fragmented.

In Mountain View individuals moved in and out of leadership positions as and when they used cigarettes as a medium of exchange. On the other hand, there were more marked leaders in Greentrees. For example, Robert tended to answer for Richard and Howard, and Edward 'watched out' for Matthew and Frederick. Moreover, some residents in Greentrees had marked disabilities. For example, Richard had speech problems and Frederick was blind. Robert and Edward's leadership behaviours were a response to this as much as anything else.

Finally, Jane made it clear that she preferred the company of women to men. However, with the uneven distribution of female and male residents the possibility of more female company was remote:

Jane: The residents are all men aren't they? We're the only two ladies, the others are men. It would be nice to have another lady to have as a friend here.

To sum up this section, relationships between residents appeared to be based on two characteristics described in Chapter 6: hospital histories and the exchange of cigarettes. Poverty may be added to these since the exchange of cigarettes was in the main due to the inability of residents properly to fund their habit. The provision of cigarettes appeared to be the only channel through which individuals could establish a position of status and the only aspect of their lives where they were able to exert some degree of control over others.

At the same time, other residents of like experience were not necessarily the people with whom individuals always wanted to associate. The movement from hospital to the community was without a doubt a major life change for residents. To a degree this was cushioned by sharing the same life space with others who share in a common predicament.

Social acquaintances and social support

There were individuals in both projects who reported that they would like to meet 'new friends' but very few residents had network members not associated with the psychiatric system. Those who expressed a desire to meet people away from their residences also felt that they had 'more in common' with 'ordinary' people. This was particularly true for Robert who interacted with members of his local choir and

David who had made friends with a few individuals in local cafés. Since these individuals regarded their fellow residents to be 'mentally ill' their own association with people who were not ill reinforced their own identity of being 'well' and 'normal'.

Characteristics unique to certain individuals facilitated their contacts with social acquaintances. For instance, Robert's ability to sing and speak Welsh meant that he could participate in particular local activities like the choir. Similarly, David's enjoyment and ability to communicate on a wide range of subjects meant that he could very easily talk to many different people. Given the significant negative link ($r=-0.6$ $p<.01$) between General Behaviour Scores (which included speech skills and speech disturbance) and network size (using participant observation scores) and also a significant negative correlation ($r=-0.5$ $p< 0.5$) between General Behaviour Scores and number of social acquaintances, the indications are that those with poor behaviour, including communication deficits, were less likely to have social acquaintances.

Nevertheless, in Mountain View residents including Sarah, Paul, Gareth, Albert and Peter expressed their frustration at not having the opportunity to meet new people. They stated that the main reason for this was their relative financial poverty which directly affected their ability to go out and 'have a drink'.

Of those who had contact with social acquaintances, the support appeared to be multiplex (multi-stranded), involving material support (in Robert's case lifts in the car from choir practice and in David's case the exchange of cigarettes) and also confiding or conversational companionship. These relationships were formed largely as a result of the individual's own initiative and contacts generally occurred in community locations. Robert for example:

> I've met this man. He's always outside his house. He lives just down the road and stands in his garden. I've made friends with him. He's one of the residents in Small Market. I meet him quite often like. I've only known him since I've been here.

It seemed to be the case that such naturalistic settings, being free from the watchful eyes of staff, produced an environment more conducive to the formation of confiding or valued relationships with neighbours and other community members. The extent to which such relationships were of significance to residents was difficult to gauge since some were reluctant to talk about their social acquaintances. David, for example, did not wish to talk about his social acquaintance since she was a married woman and he did not want 'to put her in an awkward position by talking about her'. Nevertheless, fieldwork observations confirming residents' verbal reports also indicated that such contacts were very important to their own identities as 'ordinary' people in the community.

Service contacts and social support

In both housing projects contacts with people in their local community roles like shop keepers, waiters and waitresses, milkmen, postmen and bank managers, referred to here as service contacts, were few and far between. There was less than one such contact per individual on average. Individuals in Greentrees named more than those in Mountain View which was surprising as Mountain View was situated on the main high street in Castleton.

At the heart of this was not so much the opportunity for conversation but rather the interest in individuals shown by these significant others. Albert, for example, stated that the bank manager was important to him as '...he talks to me and sends me letters'. Even though these letters were of the formal administrative type, the receiving of such a letter was significant to Albert in the absence of any other correspondence. Similarly, Sarah stated that she was 'pleased that they all know me in the shops now. They always say hello and call me by name and we have a little chat... yes I've been really surprised'.

Interaction with people in community service roles was valued in giving individuals a sense of their own community presence, yet ties with such community members were limited. David was the only resident at Mountain View who had developed relationships with members of the community which were not based on anything other than sharing each other's lives. The first of these relationships had been initiated by a member of the service sector and is explained using the following field notes:

> David was in the café. He smiled and said 'Hello'. He took my tray to the table for me.
>
> Waitress: Give the lady the extra tea bag David.
>
> David sat down by another ex-patient and talked. The waitress joined in. David and his companion left separately at 12.45 p.m. David asked the waitress about the 'special' and said he might have it later. He said goodbye.
>
> Waitress to fieldworker: Me and David are good mates. He's a heck of a nice bloke you know. He used to come in when we had the other shop up town. I knew him when he was ill you know. He had depression and a kind of nervous breakdown. But you wouldn't know him now. There's nothing wrong with him...

In Greentrees, a local shop near to where six residents lived provided a setting in which individuals could meet workers. The proprietors and waitresses of local cafés in Small Market had soon become accustomed to their new customers. James of 'Cliffton' also stated that he often chatted to the postman, milkman and taxi driver. However, prompting revealed that unlike David's friend in the café, ties with these service contacts were weak and involved little more than passing conversations about the weather. Nevertheless, the strength of such weak ties (Granovetter, 1982) lies in their function of providing companionship, albeit for a short period of time, and giving residents a sense of sharing in community life.

However, there were also confrontations between a few residents in Mountain View and service sector contacts as the fieldnote below indicates:

> A workman came into the flat and Gareth asked him for a cigarette. The workman said 'no' as he had given him three already. Gareth swore at him and the man got upset and left. The workman then returned and told me that he felt bad but that he'd given Gareth cigs before.

Similarly, Paul was asked on numerous occasions to leave a local café due to his incessant smoking and failure to use the ash tray. For these individuals, life in community settings such as cafés and public houses was often punctuated by battles with proprietors due to the manifestation of behaviours acquired in long-stay hospital such as smoking others' discarded cigarette ends and chain smoking without adequately using ash trays. This in turn led to disappointments for individuals like Paul who desperately wanted to be part of the local community as:

> I had to leave the café, you know because they didn't like me... they didn't like me smoking you know. I smoke you see and they didn't like it. I suppose I could try going again... do you think I could go back? I could I suppose...

Relationships between residents and service contacts could therefore either be very successful, as in the case of David of Mountain View and residents in Greentrees, or could lead to frustrations for all concerned as in the case of Paul. It appeared that support with residents' social skills would go some way towards mediating interactions with members from the service sector.

Discussion

Whilst Greentrees residents construed some support from staff to be rather more characteristic of informal relations, relationships were still perceived in terms of the medical model with degrees of social distance between staff and residents. However, people's personal histories were also implicated in these perceptions. Longitudinal study would be necessary to see whether, with the passage of time, these relationships become less formal. Similarly, in Mountain View where the family model of care was not in evidence, residents generally perceived project workers as similar to hospital staff. Key worker arrangements providing for greater continuity in relationships were helping to create possibilities for more person-centred support and closer, more personal relationships with residents. However, the 'popular patient' syndrome was still in evidence, to a degree reflecting people's compliance with house rules. Maintenance of good relationships with staff was therefore dependent upon patronage of the rules of the game. Rehabilitative prospects for unpopular residents were therefore not good.

The different value positions regarding contact with kin are interesting, reflecting on the one hand unfulfilled expectations about more contact, and on the other hand anxieties about receiving visits which would serve to remind individuals about their dependent status. Despite having moved on from hospital, some residents still equated their place of residence with that of a mental health establishment which they did not want family members to visit.

There were few outlets for residents to express themselves either through valued occupational or social roles. Relationships with other residents could be very exploitative and based, almost wholly in some cases, on bartering for cigarettes. Although many natural friendships had formed between residents, some individuals were seen to withdraw in order to disassociate themselves from those similarly labelled as 'mentally ill'. This basic contradiction in people's perceptions would seem to warrant further consideration by policy makers and service planners.

Relationships with community members including social acquaintances and service sector members were found to be sparse but still meaningful to those concerned. In particular, residents enjoyed others' interest in their lives. Residents in Greentrees appeared to have more opportunities to meet community members since staff structured their days to incorporate outings into the local town. Whilst the residents of Mountain View appeared to long for relationships with 'ordinary' people, and tried their best to integrate, they often lacked the social skills necessary to be accepted by local people. The result was too often disappointment and rejection.

The salience of structured care practices underlined by a clear philosophy of direct care is highlighted. How support provided can mediate mental health, social functioning and social integration is the subject of the next chapter.

Summary

- Relationships with staff could be characterised along a formal-informal care continuum. For some residents, staff were playing out roles which reinforced social distancing. House rules were used as a means to reinforce compliance and one's acceptability or popularity with staff could depend upon patronage of such rules. To a degree key worker systems were allowing more personal relationships to be fostered with staff.
- Some individuals wanted more contact with family members. Phone calls and letters could have special significance when visits from families were infrequent or difficult. It appeared to be difficult to organise visits by residents to families.
- Other individuals wished to avoid further physical contact with family members, ostensibly because they thought it would add to the weight of family

obligations or because visits by families to their adopted home would remind them of their perceived status as labelled persons.

- There were similarly ambivalent attitudes about fostering close relationships with other residents. Common histories united some individuals and allowed friendships to grow but in other cases prompted withdrawal and rejection.
- Dependency on the cigarette sub-culture led to some exploitative relationships between residents.
- People's acquired social skills and cultural affinities predisposed to the development of relationships with a variety of people, neighbours and those in service roles, in the community.

9 Outcomes of community care

> You feel much better being out of hospital. You feel like you are chained up and when you go out you are free, free as a bird.
>
> Robert

An attempt is made in this chapter to investigate the relationships between outcomes for individuals and their support network characteristics. The outcomes of concern here are mental health, social functioning and social integration. It is hoped that the analysis will provide some indication of how social networks and social support function to aid successful adjustment to life in the community.

Mental health, social functioning and social integration - interrelated outcomes?

Studies which assess outcomes for individuals discharged from long-stay hospitals have traditionally indicated an association between clinical and social functioning and integration (TAPS, 1990; Melzer et al. 1991). Reports of successful outcomes have linked fewer psychiatric symptoms and fewer hospital re-admissions with better living and social skills and more social contacts (Stein and Test, 1980; Hoult et al. 1981). Similarly, studies which show little overall improvement in outcomes again indicate an association between the three variables (Marks, 1992). In particular, having fewer friends has been related to poorer psychiatric outcomes (Strauss and Carpenter, 1972) and improved social networks associated with better social functioning (Thornicroft and Breakey, 1991).

However, more recent research suggests a divergence of psychiatric and behavioural outcomes (Anderson et al. 1993). For example, Reda (1994) found some deterioration in patients' mental state six and twelve months post-discharge but improvements in hygiene standards, social networks and attitudes towards community living. Perkins et al. (1992) described how, two months after hospital discharge, individuals showed no deterioration in REHAB disturbed speech measures despite an increase in active psychotic symptoms. Similarly, although Holloway and Faulkner (1994) found no evidence of an improvement in the underlying psychiatric illnesses of their study group following discharge, modest gains in social functioning were observed.

With the aforementioned findings in mind, the relationships between the three outcome measures were examined. Described in detail in Chapter 3, Krawiecka Rating Scale scores (KRS) were used as a measure of psychiatric state, and REHAB Total General Behaviour Scores (TGBS) as an indication of social functioning. The more complex concept of social integration was measured in terms of three dimensions: (i) participation in community activities; (ii) community network membership; and (iii) perceived social integration. These are described in more detail later. However, briefly stated, participation in community activities refers to individual involvement in community life such as voluntary work, sport and local entertainment. The number of community activities in which individuals were involved was scored. Community network membership relates to the number of network members who are from the local community but not connected to psychiatric services. Finally, perceived social integration refers to whether or not individuals perceive themselves to be socially integrated within the community. Affirmative and negative answers were scored.

Using the Wilcoxon sign test a significant difference ($p<.001$) was found between psychiatric state and social functioning. These findings suggest that the performance of basic living and social activities for independent community living are unrelated to psychiatric symptomatology. This supports Vitalo (1971), Englehardt and Rosen (1976) and Cohen and Anthony (1984) who argue that measures of psychiatric symptoms do not correlate with living, social and vocational skills.

There was a reasonably close association between participation in community activities and community network membership ($r=0.5$ $p<.05$). This was expected since community activities provide contexts within which community network members including service contacts and social acquaintances may be reached. However, neither of these variables were in turn associated with perceived social integration.

No statistical relationship was found between psychiatric state and the three measures of social integration. Hence the link between community integration and psychiatric state previously reported in the literature (Dayson, 1992; Thornicroft and Breakey, 1991) does not characterise this study group. Rather, it suggests that community integration is not contingent upon the absence or reduced level of psychiatric symptomatology.

Significant negative associations between TGBS and scores for participation in community activities ($r=-0.45$, $p<.05$) suggest that poor living and social skills are linked to participation in fewer social activities, supporting the idea that social and living skills are necessary for engaging in community pastimes such as recreational and work orientated activities (Anthony and Liberman, 1986). A significant negative correlation was also found between TGBS and community network membership ($r=-0.46$, $p<.05$) indicating an association between social functioning and at least two measures of social integration. This lends some support for the idea that social functioning may be a necessary conduit towards social integration. TGBS scores and perceived social integration were however unrelated.

These statistically based findings suggest that psychiatric state bears little relationship to how people function socially. They further support the view that social functioning has different implications for different aspects of social integration. This is explored further by examining how social network characteristics and social support might mediate different outcomes for individuals.

Social networks, social support and mental health revisited

In Chapter 1 it was argued that social networks and social support can play a significant role in mediating mental health (Pattison, 1977; Cohen and Sokolovsky, 1978a, 1979; Eisemann and Perris, 1985; Kinard, 1995). However, it has also been suggested that how an individual construes their network relationships and support provided is more important to mental health than the presence of relationships and support (Henderson, 1985; Eurelings-Bontekoe et al. 1995).

In seeking to link social networks with mental health, studies have tended to emphasise the structural aspects of networks (Segal and Holschuh, 1991) but have taken different positions regarding the most optimal network types. Some argue that large social networks are associated with happiness, well-being and mental health (Pattison et al. 1975; Cohen and Sokolovsky, 1978b) despite their composition (Burt, 1987; Acock and Hurlbert, 1990) or interactional characteristics (Gerstel et al. 1985). By contrast, others argue that smaller networks (Taylor et al. 1984) of high density and homogenous nature (Walker et al. 1977) are more supportive during crisis periods than wide, dispersed networks (Caplan, 1974). However, Cotterill (1994) qualifies this point by stating that such a network type may only be therapeutic if the social costs of interacting with others are minimised, thereby protecting against over-stimulation (ibid, p.125) since social relationships can be the sources of strain and may mediate conflict as well as support (Rook, 1990; Acock and Hurlbert, 1990; Samter, 1994; Ell, 1996).

Strong, close ties as well as the supportive function of confiding have been posited as the key interactive dimensions of social networks (Brown and Harris, 1978) and the presence of a confidant within one's social network has been linked to prevention and improvement of mental health disorders including clinical depression (Surtees, 1980; Gottlieb, 1985; Paykel et al. 1980) and schizophrenia (Turner, 1979).

Brown and Harris (1978) also found different types of social support to be important for different diagnostic groups. Furthermore, Breier and Strauss (1984) reported that individuals found different types of help to be relevant to different phases of their recovery from psychotic episodes. Ventilation, reality testing, social approval and integration, material support, problem solving and constancy were reported as the most commonly named functions. These were also described as being the most useful during convalescence from psychotic episodes whilst motivation, reciprocal relating and symptom monitoring were reported as most conducive to the rebuilding phase of illness (see Breier and Strauss, 1984, p.952-953).

Cotterill (1994) argues that very small networks may only be beneficial if they provide flexible support during different phases of psychiatric illness, but that they are more likely to be insufficient for the needs of people with schizophrenia in terms of the amounts of social support or social control they provide. She qualifies this by linking the involvement of the young, single males in her study who experience the 'revolving door' pattern of care with the impoverished nature of their social networks which may have been insufficient for their social support needs (ibid, p.26).

Little attention appears to have been given to identifying the specific qualitative factors within a social relationship that might prove useful for patients recovering from mental illnesses (Leavy, 1983; Breier and Strauss, 1984). Accordingly, relationships between types of support and psychiatric state need to be subjected to further examination.

Residents' perceptions of factors mediating mental well-being

Analysis of case study data made it possible to examine the qualitative aspects of social relationships, as construed by individuals themselves, for their association with psychiatric illnesses. This follows Breier and Strauss (1984) whose work appears to suggest that different aspects of social relationships are helpful to persons with psychiatric disorders. These however need to be tested empirically.

During interviews there was an opportunity to ask individuals about the extent to which they felt that relocation into the community and consequent social support had mediated their own mental health. The strength of this line of investigation is that it begins to define the world as the individuals themselves see it. At the same time it has to be appreciated that the connections which individuals make between support in the community and mental health offers only one perspective, and one in which there are vested interests.

Perceived improvement in mental health appeared to be dependent upon how individuals defined their mental state. This was not necessarily synonymous with their clinical diagnosis or their KRS score. Six residents in Mountain View (Sarah, Albert, Gareth, Saul, David and Peter) stated that they did not have schizophrenia as diagnosed but suffered from either 'depression', 'epilepsy', 'mental disorder', 'had rebelled against society' or 'had recovered' from mental illness.

For those four residents who did not express disagreement with their diagnostic label, they each stated that they felt 'much better' living in the community. However, only two residents in Mountain View equated this with support provided as well as their renewed independence. Chris indicated that household support as well as decision-making and feedback made a difference to his mental health:

> I prefer it here. I'm still on all the pills but feel better you know. I think it's because I am more independent - here you do things for yourself but the staff, they look after my affairs, my money and things... and help me to cook and things you know.

On the other hand, Paul and Daniel were unable to explain what it was that helped them feel better mentally. Residents in Greentrees also found difficulties in explaining how social support might aid their mental state. This was again due in part to their poor communication skills but also, in the case of Richard and Sidney, to their expressed view that the subject of their mental health was 'the doctor's job' rather than theirs to comment upon.

Nevertheless, those who were able to express a point of view about their mental health (N=7/15) all stated that they 'felt better living here' and linked this improvement in health to household support as well as to material support, stating they were 'better looked after' in the community than in hospital and that they had 'more freedom'.

Further mediating factors for individuals' mental health apart from household and material support reported by residents included confiding, decision-making and feedback, and surveillance. These are discussed in more detail below.

Confiding and mental health

Individual scores for psychiatric state provided scope to examine the association between having a confidant, number of confidants and psychiatric state (measured using KRS) six months after hospital discharge. Firstly, comparative analysis was achieved by splitting the cohort (N=25) into those who had confidants (N=11) and those who did not (N=14). Since numbers were small, and there was missing KRS data for three residents, the raw data for both variables were analysed.

There was an observed difference in psychiatric state between those individuals who had confidants and those who did not (mean raw KRS scores of 12% and 16% respectively), suggesting some marginal evidence that the presence of a confidant may be linked to better mental health. On the other hand, whilst there were only five individuals with confidants (33%) in Greentrees as opposed to seven in Mountain View (70%), in Greentrees there was no difference in psychiatric state between those who had confidants and those who did not (both having a mean score of 16%). This implies that for individuals in Greentrees, having a confidant made little difference to their mental health whilst within Mountain View the presence of a confidant was associated with a difference, individuals with confidants having a mean score of 10 per cent whilst those without had a mean score of 16 per cent. The mean number of confidants for residents in Greentrees (0.26) was less than for those in Mountain View (1.4). Although Greentrees residents had poorer speech skills than Mountain View residents a significant negative correlation between speech skills or speech disturbance and number of confidants in a person's support network was not found. Other explanations for individual differences in the number of confidants were therefore explored.

Correlations between network size and number of support types with number of confidants per person ($r=0.4$ $p<.05$) ($r=0.5$ $p<.01$) were statistically significant. Larger networks and more support types were therefore associated with having more confidants. This is one possible explanation as to why Mountain View residents had more confidants than those at Greentrees. Nevertheless, whilst larger networks and more support types are associated with more confidants, there was found to be no observed or statistical link between the number of confidants a person had and their psychiatric state. Instead it is the presence of a confidant rather than the number of confidants which is linked to better psychiatric outcome.

That having a confidant was important to individuals' perceptions of mental health was illustrated by Sarah and Chris:

Sarah: ... well I can talk to my friend (hospital contact). I trust and confide in her. You have to have someone like that, don't you, to help you? If I'm feeling depressed and I'm crying, she helps me and I help her as well.

Observations of Sarah and her friend substantiated Sarah's comment. Her friend was often to be seen in the communal lounge of Mountain View comforting Sarah who was in an obvious state of depression, whispering to her, asking if she was 'alright' and 'what's wrong?' The two friends would then decide on where to go 'for a chat' and would leave for either Sarah's flat or a café in Castleton.

Chris: I trust my keyworker and another woman. She was the decorator's daughter but she works in a hostel now. I can confide in her. I tell her my thoughts and she helps my mind.

Similarly, Saul stated that he often 'felt better' after he had spoken to Chris whom he found he could talk to about his inner thoughts and feelings. Confiding or being able to 'talk to' a confidant is close to the idea of 'ventilation' described by Breier and Strauss (1984) as a means of reducing anxiety and tension and making patients 'feel better' (ibid, p.950). Samter (1994), in a study of lonely students, similarly points to the positive results of emotional acceptance and/or reassurance from the communicative capacity of network members. For the residents in this study, confiding was adjudged important to a sense of mental well-being.

Decision making, feedback and mental health

Seven residents in Mountain View including those who did not express strong negative opinions about their psychiatric label (Jane, Chris, Paul and Daniel) described how 'decision-making and feedback' helped them 'feel better mentally'.

Sarah stated that she received feedback from staff concerning thoughts such as 'when I think that someone is after me' or when she was 'distressed' at which times staff would tell her that she was imagining things and/or would comfort her by 'talking to' her. Another example of the positive effect of feedback was when she thought that 'people were coming out of the clock' in her lounge until staff reassured her that she had imagined it. Similarly, the police station across the road from Mountain View was often visited by Sarah during episodes of paranoia. At these times the police would provide feedback as to whether events were real or imagined. Such interactions between Sarah and people in her support network helped her to distinguish between reality and her psychotic distortions.

Other individuals such as Chris and Paul were observed to 'test out' ideas and behaviour on staff. Chris often talked about his past cricket friends as though they existed in the present and staff would consequently endeavour to put him right on this account. Similarly, Paul and Gareth would engage in behaviour likely to result in a reaction from staff and would look 'over their shoulders' to observe the response. Such behaviour included looking down chairs and in bins for cigarettes and, for Paul, taking alternate steps on the pavement, or standing in the middle of the street praying. Responses from staff were erratic. Sometimes they corrected Paul and Gareth and sometimes they did not, in the belief that the residents should 'learn by themselves what is acceptable and what is not in society'.

Decision-making and feedback from staff therefore provided residents with an opportunity to engage in 'reality testing'. 'Reality testing' as a helpful function of social relationships was also described by Breier and Strauss (1984). In their study of patients 12 months post-hospital discharge after a psychotic episode, 5/20 described how within the context of social relationships they distinguished the boundaries of reality and tested delusional thoughts through feedback from others.

Albert expressed the view that he 'felt better' mentally since he had been encouraged by staff and fellow colleagues to be the residents' representative. He argued that this had been beneficial to him since it was one way in which he could prove to himself that he could handle things on his own. Residents all too infrequently had the opportunity to take on responsibilities in this way but when in Albert's case it did happen the difference to his self-esteem was obvious.

Linked to the lack of roles and responsibilities for individuals were feelings of boredom. Whilst Albert was able to assume a leadership role this was intermittent and limited to monthly staff-resident meetings. In the main he argued that 'I get bored sitting back doing nothing' and that this made him 'suffer'. Similarly, Gareth equated boredom with feeling unwell:

> I feel terrible. I'm not well... it's boring here, there's nothing to do. I get bored...

Likewise, in the day-to-day book, a comment referring to David also implied that boredom did little for mental health:

Day-to-day 23 May 1991. Mood down - could be that he's bored? Not doing enough to occupy his mind?

As stated earlier the philosophy of Mountain View prevented staff from making decisions or instructing residents on how to structure their day. It is plausible that such behaviour could have helped individuals had it been provided.

Structured activities or 'having something to do' has been cited in the literature as fundamental to improvement in psychiatric illness (Dincin, 1975; Brabbins et al. 1995). Structured activities such as arts, crafts and exercises have been found to lead to a significant reduction in bizarre behaviours such as inappropriate laughter or mumbling to self (Wong et al. 1986). Breier and Strauss (1984) also argued that the encouragement to achieve higher levels of occupational and social functioning was important to recovery from a psychotic disorder. Residents in Mountain View had very few structured activities available to them and it seems clear that it was one of the contributory reasons for poor psychiatric symptomatology among residents there.

Surveillance and mental health

Residents such as Frederick and Matthew who knew that fellow colleagues and staff were 'watching out' for their well-being stated that they 'felt better knowing someone cared about them' and were 'seeing that they were alright'. This ties in with previous research which suggests that perceived support is linked to mental health (Eurelings-Bontekoe et al. 1995).

On the other hand, individuals with symptoms of paranoia resented such intrusion. Sarah, for example, asked 'why do the staff keep staring at me all the time? I don't like it', highlighting the potential problems of surveillance if not carried out sensitively. The iatrogenic effects of support on symptomatology have already been documented (Johnstone, 1993; Ell, 1996).

Comment

This exploratory analysis has presented some indications about how different types of support may mediate feelings of psychiatric well-being. The findings, though only tentative and impressionistic, point to the importance of confiding, decision-making and feedback, and surveillance to an understanding of psychiatric state. These types of support appear to have parallel functions to those of reality testing, motivation, problem solving, and ventilation described by Breier and Strauss (1984) which are reported to mediate mental health.

Social networks, social support and social functioning - an investigation

Social functioning is defined as a rehabilitated 'state' in which individuals, using functional skills, are able to interact with others in a way that is meaningful to them and in which they may enjoy and socially participate in recreational activities without feeling isolated or lonely - factors also necessary for the 'state' of social integration. An analysis of possible links between individuals' social networks, social support and social functioning (measured by using Rehabilitation Hall and Baker (REHAB - Total General Behaviour Scores, TGBS)) is presented below.

For the study group as a whole there was found to be a significant negative link between network size and TGBS ($r=-0.6$, $p<.01$), implying that opportunities to interact with more network members are associated with better social functioning. With individuals in Mountain View having larger networks, it would be assumed that they would also have lower (better) general behaviour scores than their Greentrees counterparts. However, as indicated in Chapters 3, 4 and 6, residents in Greentrees had fewer network members but lower general behaviour scores than residents in Mountain View. Further analysis found a significant negative link between the number of social acquaintances in a person's network and TGBS scores ($r=-0.50$, $p<0.5$). This is salient because no significant associations were found between TGBS scores and the number of people in the other network membership groups. The networks of Mountain View residents comprised mostly other residents and hospital contacts (46.5%) compared to Greentrees (37.4%) (Forrester-Jones and Grant, 1995). Therefore, Mountain View residents were generally associating with others who had similar problems of social functioning to themselves. Previous literature has commented that such association is likely to reinforce behaviour reminiscent of the psychiatric sub-culture (Caudhill, 1958; Estroff, 1985; Barham and Hayward, 1991; McCourt Perring, 1993).

The associated longitudinal investigation by Crosby and Barry (1995) mapped total general behaviour by time spent in the community. At hospital baseline, Greentrees residents were found to have had worse TGBS scores than their colleagues in Mountain View, (mean=61.92 and 30.64 respectively) explained as due to differences in age (Greentrees being older) and varying lengths of hospitalisation (Crosby et al. 1995a). Whilst all residents were found to show marked improvements in relation to social activity, level of self-care, community and speech skills (ibid), at six weeks and six months post-discharge, differences between projects were found to have diminished significantly (Crosby et al. 1995a).

Assessment at 12 months post-discharge showed that total general behaviour scores for residents in Mountain View had significantly deteriorated to a score of 42.07 ($p<.01$) whereas the TGBS score for Greentrees had significantly improved to 44.34 ($p<.01$) (Crosby et al. 1995a). Explanations for this included an increased staff-client ratio as well as a care management philosophy and practice in Greentrees which emphasised participation (ibid). The study reported a significant link between the simple separate main effect of relocation and TGBS scores for Greentrees ($p<.002$) but no significant result for Mountain View ($p<.095$) (ibid, p.99).

The social functioning of residents in Greentrees had therefore improved more than those in Mountain View, despite the fact that they had fewer network members. Whilst longitudinal data for individuals was not available in this study, the types of support described in Chapter 7 were analysed in an attempt to identify whether they were associated with social functioning.

Cross-tabulations were computed for possible links between TGBS scores and support types. Non significant links were found between TGBS and household support, personal support, decision making and feedback, and surveillance. Links with companionship could not be computed since all residents received this support. More significant links were expected but the small sample size reduces the discriminatory power. However, there was a significant link between TGBS and material aid (χ^2 square = 6.33, $p<.01$). One possible explanation for this was that individual factors within TGBS included social activity and community skills which, as discussed in Chapter 6, invariably required financial aid. Nevertheless, observation showed that there were some associations between social functioning and support types.

TGBS scores (as a proxy for dependency) from REHAB were examined for possible links with confiding. Individuals who had someone to confide in had lower (meaning better) TGBS (20% and 35% respectively) than those without a confidant (36% and 40% respectively), supporting the idea of a link between the existence of a confidant and lower levels of behavioural dependency.

Turning to case study material possible links between social functioning and other support types (household, personal, decision making and feedback, material aid, and surveillance) are investigated further below.

Household support and social functioning

Initial observations at the beginning of fieldwork found residents in Greentrees to be more industrious than their Mountain View counterparts in relation to their use of living skills. Only two residents from Mountain View, Sarah and Jane, had skills in cooking, budgeting, shopping, washing clothes and personal care - all associated with 'women's work'.

Whilst the eight men in Mountain View had the capacity to look after themselves, as time passed during the fieldwork period they were observed to engage less and less in the performance of living skills. Gareth, Saul and Paul put increasingly less effort into cleaning their flat and it was noticed that Gareth tended to eat uncooked food. Similarly, Saul, Daniel and, in particular, David and Peter were observed to frequent local cafés for sustenance though they occasionally asked Sarah to cook for them. Whilst eating out may be one route to social integration, it appeared to lead to failures in budgeting and in the motivation to cook for oneself. Poor budgeting resulted in further poverty which in turn led some residents to ask or beg for money and cigarettes.

A different picture emerged from observations of Greentrees. When residents were first resettled into their houses, their high level of dependence led staff to take charge of most household chores with little involvement from residents (Forrester-Jones and Grant, 1995). Nevertheless, analysis of the care practices within each house found different routines based on variants of the family model. This led to an emphasis on different aspects of living skills. In 'Hendy' a structured routine based around household chores was observed. Whilst staff provided much of the household support, room was made for residents to take responsibility for their own tasks. As a result of this Andrew hoovered every morning, Thomas helped to cook meals and desserts and both men helped in the garden..

Similarly, although staff in 'Dayspring', 'Woodlands', 'Cliffton', and 'Brangwyn' started out by providing household support, residents were allocated routine tasks (gardening, emptying the bins, bringing in the post and milk bottles, paying the milkman, laying the table, washing up and so on) which they were expected to undertake on a regular basis. Individuals became quite adept at these tasks. Whilst not being totally independent of staff, some individuals were observed to function better than some of the younger, supposedly more able residents in Mountain View.

Personal support and social functioning

As reported in Chapter 6 residents in Greentrees were observed to be cleaner and more neatly presented than those in Mountain View, showing fewer unusual traits in regard to clothes. This was viewed as a direct result of staff support. Nevertheless, interesting variations in personal presentation were observed between houses which were to a large degree due to the existence of different care practices.

In 'Dayspring', where the immediate goal was one of 'community acceptance', daily routines incorporated personal care in the form of prompting the three men to wash, shave, wear clean clothes and take pride in their appearance, to the extent of wearing colour co-ordinated garments. Observations showed that whilst staff washed and ironed clothes, the residents themselves would dress, choose what to wear, check themselves in the mirror, and take care to comb their hair before venturing out into the local town. Similarly, personal hygiene was encouraged by staff in 'Cliffton'. As the fieldwork period progressed James was observed to choose his clothes for the day and ask staff if he could buy new clothes, knowing exactly which styles and colours he wanted. On the other hand, since social integration was not significant for staff in 'Woodlands', residents were observed to be less well groomed, in some instances wearing the same clothes for several days at a time.

Whilst some residents in Mountain View such as Jane, Sarah, David and Peter evidently took pride in their personal hygiene and presentation, self care, maintenance of clothing and wearing clothes properly was a problem for the other six residents. Saul could be found walking into town only wearing trousers and shoes and Paul tended not to wash. Whilst most individuals were supposed to self-medicate, some did not, which in Saul's case precipitated re-admission to hospital. Little personal support was provided to these residents and whilst members of staff would sometimes comment upon individuals' appearance, the commitment to residents' rights to freedom of choice meant that, to a large extent, if individuals wished to wear dirty and inappropriate clothes then this was their prerogative.

Provision of personal support by staff was based upon residents' acceptance or refusal to be helped. The result was a group of individuals who appeared to have the potential to succeed in learning new and using already acquired living skills but who were not using them on an everyday basis. This deficiency was inextricably linked to the way in which household and personal support was provided. Due to the prevailing philosophy and care practices, supportive interventions were sparse and normally consisted only of a 'helping hand' now and again. Such loyalty to laissez-faire principles seemed bound to reinforce dependence.

Feedback, material aid, surveillance and social functioning

In Greentrees feedback was in evidence through prompting residents at meal times to eat properly and encouraging them to use table manners. Residents there were generally found to have good social skills. Whenever the researcher visited the houses, she was normally greeted at the door by one of the residents, welcomed, told to take her coat off and invited to have a cup of tea. Residents also answered the telephone and would ask each other if they wanted cups of tea or a snack. Greentrees staff were observed to keep a watchful eye over residents, helping them to adjust their clothes or hair so that their personal presentation conformed to normative expectations. Staff in some houses also sometimes used their own cars to take residents out to cafés, pubs and restaurants where individuals could practice their social skills. In this sense support could be construed as being a means to rehabilitative ends.

This provided a sharp contrast with Mountain View where support was more ad hoc. There, the communal lounge had more of an atmosphere akin to the hospital ward which was rather sterile. Rarely did staff help residents with their personal presentation or social skills or escort them into town. This meant that conflicts could arise when staff did accompany residents on the occasional outing. For example whilst in a café in Harlech a project worker became agitated with Paul because he slurped his tea and drank from the saucer. However, such behaviour was common to Paul when he visited local cafés. It came as a shock to him to be admonished for behaviour that was not alien to himself or the other residents.

Summary

Generally residents in Greentrees exhibited better social functioning skills than those in Mountain View. This finding appears largely to be a function of differences in care philosophies and of types of support provided. This is substantiated by the findings of the related study which also suggested links between Total General Behaviour Scores and care practices (Crosby et al. 1995b). The key factors in this may be seen to lie within an emphasis on residents' involvement in domestic routines and their responsibility for household chores.

Types of social support are also important to the achievement of social functioning outcomes. In particular, household, personal, feedback and surveillance were found to mediate Greentrees residents' development or re-development of social skills.

Social integration

This section analyses the extent to which the study group may be said to be socially integrated. Statistical analysis showed no significant links between support types and measures of integration. However, there were indications that associations between variables might be significant if the data set were larger. Nevertheless, it is hoped that the following account will provide some clues as to how social networks and social support may mediate social integration. Three further dimensions to social integration can also be discerned in the literature (Giggs, 1986; Malin, 1987; Shadish and Bootzin, 1984). For simplicity these may be termed 'locational', 'environmental', and 'participatory' social integration. Two additional facets of social integration, community network membership and valued social participation are conceptualised and measured. Whilst previous researchers have tended to concentrate on one particular dimension, it will be demonstrated using the case study data, that all dimensions are interrelated and necessary considerations for successful community re-integration of long-stay hospital psychiatric patients.

Locational integration

Malin (1987) refers to locational integration as the actual placement of individuals within community settings. Residents in this study had been relocated into respective communities and so locational integration had taken place. On the other hand, Race (1987) warns that it is a mistake to assume that physical integration is all that is needed. Nevertheless, some research within this area still appears to assume that it is (Meltzer et al. 1994).

Environmental integration

It may be argued that the 'environment' can be discussed in two ways, the actual building or physical context in which individuals live, and the wider community in which people interact.

The wider community refers to what Bloor et al. (1988) term as the 'external environment' and would include facilities and activities which community members use. In this respect, such facilities including accessible mental health care are more likely to be concentrated in urban or semi-urban areas than remote rural communities. Re-housing individuals into urban communities appears to have been a normative aspect of community care in an attempt to provide 'ordinary living' (Davey, 1994) and reflected in studies of social integration (Hare, 1956; Castle and Gittus, 1957; Giggs, 1986; Cotterill, 1994; Thornicroft and Breakey, 1991). In this respect community care in practice still has a tendency to 'urbanise care' (Moon, 1988).

Both care projects in this research were set up in close-knit semi-rural communities where all the usual facilities existed (shops, cafés, public houses, churches). In particular, Small Market, being a modest sized town, was characterised by close knit informal social networks and residents living near to the town centre were soon well known within local shops and cafés. Castleton, having accommodated the psychiatric hospital for decades, was not unused to having ex-patients living within the community. Residents in this study were placed within an environment in which social integration and positive socialisation processes within the community could take place.

Meltzer et al. (1994) advocate the utilisation of a number of self-contained units of accommodation on the same site or in close proximity in order to help individuals to blend in with the locality, as well as to help preserve existing social networks (ibid, p.269). Situated within Castleton town centre along the main high street, close to all service amenities, Mountain View was physically integrated into the community. However, two nursing homes were situated in close proximity (next door and across the road) and there was a sense of 'nursing home valley' about the location. There were also several houses nearby where other ex-patients had been relocated.

Research shows that mental health and personal well-being are associated with quality housing. Crosby (1990) states:

> architecture is a type of communication whereby messages are decoded and meanings derived by the users of buildings. Meanings may be subtle and complex with even the most mundane objects acquiring significance.

Whilst the physical layout of the flats in Mountain View had been designed to 'ensure privacy and personal space', each flat was decorated and furnished in the same colour scheme and it was noted that residents had very few possessions. Such flats were hardly typical of ordinary dwellings. Davey (1994) discusses how individuals living in flats complain of feeling remote from any community life, with no real neighbourly contacts yet at the same time lacking privacy e.g. through the absence of sound insulation (ibid, p.193).

Noise was certainly a factor which residents in Mountain View often complained about. Some residents tended to stay up all night listening to the radio or watching television, reversal of sleeping patterns being symptomatic of schizophrenia (Howe, 1995). This caused problems for fellow residents since walls were not well insulated. Peter, in particular, complained that his fellow flatmate, Daniel, 'keeps me awake all night - I can't stand it'.

Whilst the self-contained flats offered privacy and independence for some individuals, others were found to be socially isolated, spending many hours alone in their flats. Therefore, although physically placed in the community, this residence was far from a 'normal' homely environment and still reflected some features of institutional environments.

On the other hand, the physical layout of Greentrees was conducive to normal living. The accommodation was similar to that of other houses in the area. This mirrors the recent desirability of using ordinary housing that blends into the locality and minimises stigma in the practice of resettlement of long-stay psychiatric patients (Bennet, 1978; Shepherd, 1984; Garety, 1988; Perkins et al. 1992). Such housing can only facilitate rather than hinder social integration (Meltzer et al. 1994).

Participatory integration

Other studies (Katz and Lyerly, 1963; Segal and Aviram, 1978) define social integration as 'normative social behaviour', referring to aspects of so-called normal life such as employment, income and spending and social participation. Within this conceptualisation, social participation refers only to the frequency with which individuals engage in particular social activities such as using public transport or engaging in a community action group. A person may therefore be defined as socially integrated if they are involved in community activities or use community facilities on a regular basis (Shadish and Bootzin, 1984). For social integration to take place, the local environment is important as the provider of facilities/activities as the context or milieu in which participation can take place.

A checklist of 20 activities was adapted (to be more relevant to the study group) from the social activity list of Shadish and Bootzin (1984) in their comparative study of the social integration of 163 psychiatric patients living in nursing homes.

The results from the checklist (Table 9.1) indicate that residents were involved in few community activities such as voluntary work, participating in or observing collective sport or attending nightclubs and parties. Age and in some cases physical disabilities explained this. However, few residents regularly visited the cinema or the library, activities which need little physical exertion. On the other hand, all of the study group were largely involved in passive activity such as watching television with 60 per cent of Mountain View residents and 93 per cent of Greentrees residents watching television daily. This confirms the results of how residents passed their time (Chapter 6) and is similar to the findings of Shadish and Bootzin (1984) who argued that the most frequent behaviours for their study group were watching television and taking a walk. Cotterill (1994) also found that her study group in Salford spent large amounts of time 'doing nothing' and 'watching television' (ibid, p.118).

Table 9.1 also shows that individuals were limited to specific social contexts in which to meet community members such as public houses and cafés. Lack of variation in social context precluded residents from meeting more than a handful of people. However, Greentrees residents were found to have more community members than those in Mountain View and whilst this was explained in part by the social support provided it could also be linked to social context. For example, a major difference was shown between Mountain View residents and Greentrees residents in terms of who participated in paid work. The case studies revealed, however, that this was mostly tied to work in the workshop and gardens at the back of the main Mountain View building. It could not therefore be said to be strictly within the community. Similarly, Shadish and Bootzin (1984) found that out of 47 individuals who reported some employment 24 (51%) were in sheltered workshops, 23 of whom worked on the grounds of their nursing home. Nevertheless, residents in Greentrees attended educational classes or hobbies and local day centres more frequently than individuals in Mountain View. Whilst most of the people attending such activities were other members of staff and residents, it was found to be a route for individuals to meet new service contacts and make social acquaintances.

Similarly, whereas no residents in Mountain View attended religious worship weekly, over a quarter (27%) of residents in Greentrees did so. This difference was not merely indicative of residents' wishes to decline attending church services. Some Mountain View residents had unfulfilled aspirations about going to church but staff accompaniment was precluded by Mountain View's philosophy. By contrast, residents in Greentrees were actively encouraged to attend church services accompanied, as necessary, by staff. By becoming a member of the local church choir, Robert became a member of a new social group disassociated from the psychiatric services. This was found to be important to his sense of self-esteem. Robert was proud to show people photographs of himself in his surplice with his church friends. This also had 'knock-on effects' for Richard and Howard who, following Robert into attending church services, met new people themselves.

Shadish and Bootzin also found that all other behaviours were engaged in less often than once a week on the average (ibid, p.1205). Similarly, in the present study, 14 out of 20 social activities were found to be engaged in monthly or less (Table 9.1). Shadish and Bootzin concluded that chronically mentally ill patients in nursing homes seemed to be as socially integrated as chronically mentally ill patients in other settings such as group homes, and the findings here appear to substantiate this. However, whilst Shadish and Bootzin link the custodial nature of the nursing home to lack of social participation, this was not the finding here. Rather, it was linked to the character of the care philosophy espoused by the two projects.

However, analysis of scales and check lists reveals that, used alone, they are inadequate measures of social integration. The checklist of 24 social behaviours presented by Shadish and Bootzin (ibid), and adapted for this study includes 12 activities which may be done passively and in isolation (for example, 'observe sports activity', 'going to the library'). Only three activities (namely 'volunteer work', 'participation in sports' and 'playing cards or games') involve social interaction with other people. Furthermore, it may be argued that the eight interactive social behaviours mapped by Shadish and Bootzin need another network member such as a relative, friend or acquaintance as a precursor. For example, in order to 'call a friend' one would already need to have a friend. It is questionable therefore, whether a person can truly be defined as socially integrated merely by virtue of 'attending' or 'engaging' in community activities.

Table 9.1

Frequency of community activity participation

Activity	Weekly %	Monthly or less %
Voluntary work		
Mountain View	0	100
Greentrees	7	93
Paid work		
Mountain View	60	40
Greentrees	7	93
Education class or hobbies		
Mountain View	0	100
Greentrees	67	33
Day centre/community centre		
Mountain View	0	100
Greentrees	73	27
Party/disco/nightclub		
Mountain View	0	100
Greentrees	0	100
Telephone relative or friend		
Mountain View	10	90
Greentrees	0	100
Meet social acquaintance/friend		
Mountain View	40	60
Greentrees	20	80
Participate in sport		
Mountain View	20	80
Greentrees	20	80
Observe collective sport		
Mountain View	0	100
Greentrees	0	100

Watch television		
Mountain View	100	0
Greentrees	100	0
Play cards or board games		
Mountain View	20	80
Greentrees	27	73
Attend religious service		
Mountain View	0	100
Greentrees	27	73
Restaurant/public house/café		
Mountain View	90	10
Greentrees	93	7
Visit library		
Mountain View	0	100
Greentrees	20	80
Use public transport		
Mountain View	0	100
Greentrees	20	80
Visit park or zoo		
Mountain View	0	100
Greentrees	20	80
Go for walk		
Mountain View	60	40
Greentrees	53	47
Go shopping		
Mountain View	100	0
Greentrees	100	0
Go to jumble sale/car boot sale		
Mountain View	20	80
Greentrees	0	100
Visit cinema/theatre		
Mountain View	0	100
Greentrees	0	100

The social network - social integration synonym

Researchers such as Acock and Hurlbert, (1990) and Cotterill (1994) have tended to use the terms social integration and social network synonymously. Therefore, network variables such as size and density have been regarded as important measures of social integration. Acock and Hurlbert (1990) argue that social integration is structural and stress that social network size is an important indicator of social integration. Similarly, Nadel (1957) argued that the larger the network the more socially integrated the person. These conceptualisations also assume that absence of a social network results in social isolation. Furthermore, Cotterill (1994) argues that the psychiatric literature emphasises the role of social isolation rather than social integration to be a possible cause, consequence and symptom of schizophrenia (ibid, p.122).

Studies that rely on network size tend to underestimate the importance of network membership, suggesting that belonging to a social group fosters group solidarity which in turn can mediate mental health (Durkheim, 1952; Warner, 1985). On the other hand Unger and Powell (1980) argue that if a network is composed of only one type of member, for example, kin, then such singularity reflects a lack of social integration which in turn can lead to low self-esteem and depression (Pattison et al. 1979). Social network membership is therefore an important indicator of integration.

In her study of 137 ex-psychiatric patients living in Salford, Cotterill (1994) also adds the dimension of 'use of time' via time-budgets to her analysis linking variables such as gender, social class and age to network size and membership. Cotterill identified two distinctive groups of Salford residents. The group of middle aged, not-single females were the most socially integrated by virtue of having large networks with high network density comprised of a high number of kin. By contrast a group of middle aged single males were regarded as the most socially isolated as they had the smallest, lowest density networks.

However, conceptualisation and measurement relied upon large network size and density as key indicators of social integration. In the present study it has been argued that density refers to the number of individuals within a network who know each other and that high density might indicate a more homogeneous group of people who may have a shared context. For example, all members might have some connection to psychiatric services. In the case of the Salford sample, membership of middle aged not-single females included a high proportion of kin members. Such limited membership therefore indicates that the group was integrated with itself rather than with community members.

Furthermore, recorded activities and time spent did not appear to fit in with the concept of social integration. The findings showed that in terms of time spent, the most integrated group of residents, middle aged not-single females, showed a lack of sociability. None of the group spent time with a friend during the week for any social activities lasting an hour or more, and none spent any evenings outside the home for recreational purposes.

The study did not describe the social contexts within which social interactions took place apart from specifying that recreation included going to public houses and coffee bars but excluded going for walks or wandering the streets. Such information about social context could have provided valuable information about where individuals are most likely to meet people. These points highlight the absence of community within Cotterill' s conceptualisation of social integration. Finally, the study gives no indication of whether and how individuals perceived themselves to be socially integrated.

Two further dimensions of social integration accordingly need to be introduced. The first dimension is community social network membership, suggesting the idea of a community of interacting people. Identification of community network members other than those associated with psychiatric services gives an indication of the extent to which individuals are interacting and integrating within that body of people. This highlights the importance of the existence of social networks and the variation of social network membership. It may be argued that network membership and participation in community social activities are closely linked since community activities provide community contexts for community members to become part of an individual's social network. Secondly, of equal importance is valued social participation and the feelings individuals have about the notion of community membership. Without understanding these perceptions social integration is in danger of being only partially operationalised. Valued social participation implies an evaluative dimension derived from the appraisals of those being studied.

Social integration via community network members

In Chapter 6, it was shown that the study group had few community members in their social networks (mean=2.1). However, community members including service contacts and social acquaintances formed a larger percentage of Greentrees residents' networks than for residents in Mountain View (15.3% and 4.8% respectively), these differences having been explained by individual and group characteristics and by contrasting care practices in the houses.

It was argued that whilst most of the study group were hindered by their psychiatric background, poverty, smoking, personal presentation and communication, staff support provided in Greentrees had at least moved some way towards alleviating some of these negative characteristics. In particular, personal and household support improved personal presentation. Opportunities to practice acquired social skills were also observed when staff encouraged residents to interact with service contacts such as milkmen, postmen and shopkeepers. By contrast the laissez-faire philosophy of Mountain View left residents to initiate relationships with community members. Support provided predominantly by other residents was not geared towards the re-acquisition of skills necessary for this. Despite some exceptions, many individuals' social lives were far from integrated with the local community judged by network membership alone. However, this begs questions about whether individuals considered themselves to be socially integrated.

Valued social participation

Valued social participation has been defined by Flynn and Nitsche (1980) as the ability and opportunity to integrate in a way that is meaningful and valuable to the individual. With this in mind it was felt to be essential to understand from the point of view of residents themselves how social integration was construed, the extent to which it was valued and whether or not they felt that their own social integration had occurred with community relocation.

What emerges is a range of views between residents regarding definitions of social integration. On the one hand, some individuals defined the issue in terms of physical and environmental integration, linking their relocation into 'normal' community accommodation with renewed community membership:

Andrew: I live in a normal ordinary place. I'm the same as everyone else. I listen to the wireless.

Sidney: I'm just like all the other people. I live here in this house - here in Small Market like.

Physical and environmental integration were also linked with issues of freedom and personal space. Ownership of privacy and independence were found to be valued by all residents, something also reported by Crosby et al. (1995b). It was felt that the physical environment and social milieux of Greentrees provided opportunities for individuals to meet others in the community. For example:

Robert: I feel I'm the same as everyone else in Small Market. I wasn't very settled there in hospital. There is more freedom here. You can please yourself where to go. You feel much better being out of hospital. You feel like you are chained up and when you go out you are free, free as a bird. I've got my independence. I can come and go as I like. I'm getting to know the people in town now.

Albert: This is a lot more of a home than at the hospital. There is more freedom to move and living in one's own apartment is good. There is more privacy here because you had to stay with that many people in the hospital. In the hospital you had three other people beside you in the ward but here we have our own rooms. In the hospital there was lots of space but they held us back from using it. It wasn't that we had freedom. It was made that you had to get consent but it's like freedom is your personal property here. I've certainly got a better chance of meeting up with these other people in Castleton. When you go along the avenues, you meet people - you seem to crash into them.

On the other hand, residents such as Chris defined social integration more directly as socialising with other residents:

Chris: I feel more integrated here. Gareth comes for a coffee and I'm more independent.

Interestingly, most residents perceived social integration to mean socialising with community members and appeared to have more of an understanding of this desired outcome of community care than staff, some of whom as already stated equated social integration with physical placement. Residents' views are illustrated well in the following quotes:

Paul: I'm reinstated in Castleton now. I have more friends and more money. I have a purpose here and I've got more freedom.

Robert: I've met someone in Small Market, he's always outside the house. I've made friends with him, he's one of the residents in Small Market. As you go down the road well he lives next to it in a cul-de-sac. I meet him quite often like. I've only known him since I've been here.

Sarah: Oh I love it here. I know all the people in the shops now.

R: Do you?

Sarah: Yeh, most of them, when I go round, call me Sarah now.

R: Really?

Sarah: Yeh. I've been quite surprised and in the [public house], they always say hello to me. I know most of them in there and I always say hello and they never pass me... I feel part of Castleton now. Oh yes, yes, oh yes I'm integrated here. I'm a member of the community and Mountain View has got me away from the hospital or I would have still been up there. It's a lovely shopping area. Umm, it reminds me of when I used to walk down from my own home, going to shops on my own, doing bits of shopping and walking back to my house. I had a lot of independence when I did that. But in the hospital you used it all. I mean you went from the hospital for a few hours to town and then thought 'oh I've got to trudge up that hill back up there' and you always had that stigma of 'I've got to go back to there'. But the stigma has lifted since I've been here. Yeh oh yeh, definitely lifted yes. Yes I do feel one of the Castleton people now. I feel like I did when I was at home like an outpatient. I used to come into the hospital but I used to come only for three months and then go home. I feel like that... umm, but a bit better, better umm... 'cos I've got me independence and I can come and go as I like and eh I don't depend on the hospital any more.

Whilst individuals valued the friendships they had made in the community, not all felt they had many opportunities to become socially integrated. In Mountain View residents regarded any strides towards social integration to be a product of their own will or initiative rather than the result of actions taken by staff. This confirms the findings reported in Chapter 5 about the care practices of staff at Mountain View. Another comment from Sarah highlights how some residents were left to themselves:

R: Do you get an opportunity to get to know people in the community?

Sarah: Umm, no not really, not much, only when I'm shopping or if I go to the hairdressers or if I go to the [public house] or if I go to the cafés in town. It's up to me. Somebody might say 'hello' and I'll sit down and say 'oh hello' and get involved with the conversation and if they don't then well I just think I'll get on with what I'm doing.

This illustrates that social integration, if left to individuals themselves, will ultimately depend upon personalities and individual preference. Sarah, being gregarious, would be more likely to meet new people than, for example, Owain who was shy and retiring. Nevertheless, whatever the personality, it was clear that some residents felt that they definitely were not socially integrated and that this was something to do with the degree of support received from network members. Interestingly, these individuals were all from Mountain View:

Gareth: Oh I don't know anybody in Castleton. I know the gardener's lad, the man I worked for at the hospital. He bought me a pint one time in the, eh, [public house] but I don't know no-one. The staff, they don't do nothing for us.

Chris: There were posters put up in the lounge about the day centre in Castleton but I didn't go 'cos no one took me.

Peter: I'm getting like a cabbage. I'm not integrated at all in the community 'cos I'm still on a section. I'll be one of Castleton when I come off the medication. I'd like a home of me own in Castleton. That place (Mountain View) is not a home...

David: ...being in Mountain View - well that hasn't helped me much with integrating you know - I do that myself you know. But my friends in Castleton - well they help me you know...

Only one resident in Greentrees suggested that he would like to be more socially integrated:

Sidney: It would be good to meet more people. I just know the ones here.

Other residents in Greentrees such as Stephen, Owain, Ruth and James were content with the people they already knew and did not want to meet anyone else.

Finally, whilst social integration and its value was defined in various terms by the study group there was a sense that they appeared to be well aware of both the intrinsic and extrinsic barriers which could prevent their participation. Characteristics common to the study group such as hospital histories, medication, smoking and poverty have been discussed in Chapter 6. With adequate staff support these traits might be managed so as not to hinder individuals in their quest to become a fuller part of the community. On the other hand, to an extent extrinsic barriers were beyond both residents' and staff control. These were barriers put up by the community members themselves (some of which were alluded to in Chapter 5) - walls of prejudiced attitudes which were possibly the hardest for individuals to break down but which were nevertheless internalised by residents. Robert illustrated this poignantly when he described how he felt when locals from Small Market objected to becoming neighbours:

Robert: There's some that didn't accept, like, at first. They don't agree to it, do they? I don't think nothing of them. I wish they'd come and been through what we'd been through in hospital like. It would do them good.

In this particular instance, the neighbours included paid staff of the psychiatric services who openly ignored both residents and project workers. In this case it is a testimony, therefore, to the tenacity of residents and the ingenuity of staff support to mediate relations between locals and residents to a stage where some individuals from Greentrees are liked and respected by the community.

This section has illustrated how individuals perceive social integration in different ways, but ways that nevertheless highlight the importance of defining the term social integration multi-dimensionally. It is evident that environment, and in particular housing that is 'homely', allowing for privacy and freedom and personal space, is important to individuals' sense of being 'ordinary' and being 'just like everyone else'. Such accommodation may be viewed as a significant precursor for opportunities to socialise with others - being able to invite a friend in for tea or coffee was important for individuals' sense of independence as mastery over their own lives. Individuals also defined social integration to mean socialising with community members. Having community members in their networks went some way to enabling residents to feel they were 'a part of the community'.

Discussion

The findings described in this chapter provide some grounds for optimism about the resettlement of people with long-term mental illnesses. Firstly, they suggest that social integration is dependent more upon how individuals are able to function socially than upon psychiatric state. The statistical grounds for this conclusion are limited due to the small study sample but case material lends further weight to the underlying argument. Secondly, although social functioning was itself restricted by limited work and day opportunities and, in the case of Mountain View residents, the absence of a clear structure for managing their lives it nevertheless underlines the scope of what could yet be achieved with a little more planning and foresight.

Residents appeared to have insights not only into their state of well-being but also into what dimensions of help or support were of benefit to them. Two implications arise. Firstly, it is possible to make some tentative connections between processes and outcomes based on the accounts of service users. Lay conceptions of psychiatric well-being and measures of social functioning were seen to be mediated by different constellations of support. This suggests that support can be meaningfully targeted to achieve different outcomes which have meaning for service users. Individuals also had some clear views about factors which acted as obstacles to achieving psychiatric well-being, social functioning and social integration. Secondly, and related to the above, is further confirmation of the idea that, in this case, residents of community mental health services can be seen as 'arbiters of standards' (Twigg and Atkin, 1994). Elsewhere Williams (1995, p256) has argued that lay health beliefs and past experiences of mental health care are both crucial to the evaluation process. The case studies affirm that service users not only have something useful and relevant to say, but crucial to the way services are designed and how they can be delivered to achieve desirable ends for individuals. Hence even amongst one of society's most vulnerable groups who have spent many years in long-stay hospitals there are no grounds for treating them as passive agents devoid of insight into their own condition. If they are to be engaged as arbiters of standards then contemporary services will have to prepare themselves for some healthy criticism and re-design.

Summary

- Social functioning and social integration were found to be unrelated to psychiatric state. This suggests that, given the right kinds of social support, individuals with mental health problems have the potential to live 'ordinary lives' in the community.

- Certain forms of support were observed to mediate feelings of psychiatric well-being (including confiding, decision-making and feedback and surveillance), as well as social functioning (household, personal, feedback, material and surveillance).
- Hospital histories, medication, smoking, poverty, communication skills, limited opportunities to form relationships with community members and prejudiced attitudes from some community members were barriers to social integration.
- Residents in Greentrees were more socially integrated into their community than those in Mountain View in terms of physical and social environment, social functioning, community social network membership, participation, and from their own subjective viewpoint. Differences between projects were linked to care practices. In Greentrees structured personal and household support from staff was provided at the expense of other types of support but aid of this kind helped to mediate social integration by enabling individuals to improve personal presentation and social skills. Residents were also provided with opportunities which mediated relationships between individuals and community contacts to develop.
- The findings suggest that community social integration involves a number of conditioning factors. A social opportunity framework or social network seems necessary to provide types of support geared towards the acquisition of skills necessary for community participation. Support needs to be structured and regular rather than ad hoc and sporadic in order for social skills to be practised and instilled.
- The types of support encountered are important to an understanding of what mediates successful community care outcomes.

10 Summary and conclusions

> Community Care is a long term undertaking and there is still much to do.
>
> Virginia Bottomley (1995)

In the introduction to this book, we defined our goals in terms of (1) describing the structure of the social networks of previously hospitalised chronically mentally ill people; (2) assessing the importance of networks of relationships to individuals and their significance to personal outcomes; and (3) exploring how the philosophy and care practices in two dissimilar community housing projects mediated residents' experience of life in the community. We hope we have largely succeeded in this task. We agree with Virginia Bottomley's well publicised observation about community care that there is 'still much to do'. The question is 'what is to be done'?

What follows is a resume of the key issues to have emerged together with an attempt to distil the more important implications for policy, practice and research in community mental health services.

Social networks as restricted structures

The findings reported in Chapter 4 about the structural properties of the social networks of people with long-term mental illness corroborate other research (Dunn et al. 1990; Thornicroft and Breakey, 1991; Nelson et al. 1992) which has suggested that the size of people's social networks is, on the whole, very restricted. It was also demonstrated that the networks of the study group were high in density suggesting that individuals generally move around within very few, but well bounded, social circles. Moreover, membership of people's networks showed that almost 80 per cent comprised people who were connected to psychiatric services as staff or service users. At the same time, relocation of individuals in local community settings appeared not to have caused serious dislocation in people's social contacts and there were signs that a good number of 'old' friendships had been maintained.

Few new close or confiding relationships appeared to have been formed with persons outside mental health services. The new community living arrangements, whilst enabling people to live *in* the community, have thus far had little impact on the generation of new opportunities for the development of new friendships involving community members. This supports Dilks and Shattock (1996, p.190) who report that level of community contact appears to be unrelated to the location of residential facilities.

Involvement of kin within people's networks was very limited both in terms of membership and contact frequency. For those with kin, ambivalent attitudes about continued contact were in evidence.

The impact of care practices on social networks

To a degree the findings about the philosophy and care practices of the two community housing schemes help to explain the structure of people's networks.

The philosophy and care practices at Mountain View were aimed at following the stated preferences of residents, much in line with current policy thinking about the importance of choice to individuals. This was achieved by adopting what was described as a laissez-faire approach. This approach to managing residents, although having laudable value-driven aims, was one which lacked a clear operational structure. Some staff members admitted confusion about their roles whilst others expressed discomfort about their 'enforced' indolence. The main consequence for residents was that their daily lives were largely devoid of a recognisable structure and there was little attempt to acquaint them with rules and norms that could be construcd as culturally valued (Wolfensberger, 1983) within the community. Accordingly, staff did not see it as part of their role to mediate the establishment of new social relationships with community members or to help individuals to become re-socialised into the work ethic. Individuals were left very much to their own devices.

Staff in Greentrees were on the whole more involved in the day-to-day support, nursing and maintenance of residents on account of the age and psychiatric state of individuals. Variants of a 'family model' of care were in evidence, though there appeared to be no overarching philosophy which united the practices of the houses. Unlike their counterparts in Mountain View, staff were given no induction or continuing education connected to values or care philosophy. Hence, decisions about practices and underlying philosophy were made 'on the hoof'. What emerged were practices in which staff and residents did much together, both within and outside the houses. Because of the greater dependency needs of residents, staff also engaged in what might be termed 'protective surveillance' (Bowers, 1987) of individuals to ensure that they came to no harm. Moreover, care was orientated towards certain aspects of rehabilitation such as personal presentation and social skills which more actively mediated the fostering of contacts with community members. Staff also accompanied individuals on trips. Whilst residents were thus provided with opportunities to form relationships with people in the local community the circumstances were usually not propitious for forming long-term relationships or friendships.

Still there was no overt attempt within either community housing project to enlist the active involvement of the community. Within Mountain View this was a matter left to individual residents' own initiative. Within Greentrees, management had decided that engaging the interests of voluntary agencies in the affairs of the houses or the residents was somehow contrary to the idea of maintaining a family model of support or 'normal' living. Consequently, care *in* the community in this instance could thus be depicted in its more limited form as *care by paid staff in the community*.

One of the unanticipated consequences of the foregoing was that individuals spent a lot of time in each other's company. This had advantages and disadvantages. On the one hand it allowed friendships, not to say close and confiding relationships, to develop between individuals but on the other hand some relationships were extremely exploitative. There were also individuals who wished to disassociate themselves from other residents because of the ready attachment of an 'illness' label. The needs of such individuals were not well catered for.

Involvement in the management of homes

Different approaches to engaging residents in the management of houses was in evidence, this again being important to some understanding of how residents were assisted towards exercising choice, independence and ownership.

Within Mountain View an individual action plan and key worker systems were in operation, ostensibly to develop, maintain and monitor support tailored to the needs of the individual. Residents had access to their files and were expected to take part in decisions associated with their care plans. There was also a residents' committee which met monthly to provide an opportunity for people to raise issues of concern to themselves. Although this succeeded in the view of staff in its aim of encouraging self advocacy it did not appear to lead to the greater involvement of residents in the running of the house.

In Greentrees there was also an individual action plan system but without being linked to a formal arrangement with key workers. In the absence of such an arrangement the staff gravitated to their own informal key worker system in efforts to ensure individualised support. However, there were monthly meetings within each house which brought together staff and residents in an attempt to involve residents in the management of the affairs of the house. For a variety of reasons, including the poverty of speech of individuals, and the rather token way in which the meetings were used by staff to confirm their own ideas, neither staff nor residents attached much value to them.

However, key workers were often regarded by residents as personal confidants and this served to reinforce their perceptions of self-worth. In this sense this aspect of managing the houses contributed immeasurably to promoting independence.

Variants of a 'family model' of care were evident, reflecting not only residents' personal needs but also the different value positions taken up by staff or management about direct intervention. In regard to the evidence about social functioning and social integration it is difficult to refute the claims of the more interventionist care practice models. The laissez-faire model of Mountain View left much to be desired in this connection. However, the arrangements still fell somewhere short of enabling people to achieve a sense of ownership of the homes in which they lived. Though addressing the needs of people with severe learning disabilities, O'Brien (1994) has suggested that the right to support of individuals in their own homes involves three pre-conditions, namely that people: experience a sense of place; by themselves, or in tandem with their agent, control their home and the support necessary to live there; and experience security of place by holding the role of home owner or tenant. For most individuals the first of these pre-conditions was met but the second and third were far from being achieved. Continued residence was based very much on patronage of the 'rules'.

Whatever may be said of the philosophies and care practices of the houses, all of the residents reported that they were satisfied with their new living environment and that the 'house' was the thing they liked most about living in the community. No-one indicated a wish to return to hospital.

The struggle with identity

The accounts of residents about their daily lives and the support available to them showed them to be people with distinct personalities, life histories and lifestyles. In particular, they illustrated the importance of people and events in their lives prior to first admission to hospital. The opportunity to maintain friendships and acquaintances made in hospital enabled residents in both projects to derive the benefits of companionship when they first moved into their new community settings at a point which could otherwise have proved socially disruptive. The common bond of hospital life and experience was a subject which residents often talked about. However, as time progressed, many residents were found to become increasingly frustrated at having only 'ex-psychiatric patients' as companions. Since they were now living in the community away from the hospital, they eschewed identification of being 'ill'. Hence, individuals with such predispositions wished to associate with others who did not carry the stigma of having been hospitalised. Unfortunately, the day centres and craft clubs still offered few opportunities for individuals to meet people unconnected to the psychiatric system.

People's efforts to become comfortable with a new identity in the community were thwarted in a number of important ways. Inattention to personal presentation and social skills development left some individuals, especially those at Mountain

View, exposed to the vagaries of an impatient and sometimes hostile community in which it was almost impossible to forge long-term relationships or friendships. Prolonged hospitalisation had also left a legacy in terms of chain-smoking and lack of valued structured activity. Individuals did not know how to spend their time productively. Some even found the concept of time difficult to contend with. Besides boredom, frustration, and lowered self-image, a common consequence was relative poverty which further restricted participation in community activities. The ad hoc attempts to engage residents in 'paid' activity were token and even exploitative.

Support - a key to community care outcomes

The findings reaffirm the multi-dimensional character of support. They also illustrate how apparently mundane interactions between staff and residents can have major influences on people's self-image and conceptions of independence. Feedback and encouragement from staff and others or, to use Breier and Strauss's (1984) terms, the opportunity for residents to engage in 'reality testing', were shown to be critical influences here. However, it was not clear that this involved the multi-stage approach described by Howe (1995, pp.140-151) as comprising reassurance in the aftermath of a breakdown, dealing with lingering or persistent symptoms and just checking! Residents frequently looked to people other than staff for such feedback. Contexts where privacy was required seemed to make it possible for more confiding relationships to be established with members of staff. It was therefore rather disappointing to note the high proportion of individuals without confidants in their networks. Deficits in conversational companionship between residents were also in evidence. This had more to do with the avoidance of either exploitative relationships or association with others labelled as 'mentally ill' than with the poverty of speech of individuals. On the basis of such evidence it would have to be concluded that small group living arrangements do not eradicate problems associated with institutional life. Small-scale living does not guarantee a person-centred approach although it may in many respects make it easier to accomplish.

To a degree the individual needs of residents dictated patterns of support, the older and more disabled individuals in Greentrees receiving proportionately more personal and household assistance. However it was also interesting to observe that although they had smaller networks, residents at Greentrees were as likely to experience a diversity of support at least as great as that of their colleagues at Mountain View. In this context small and dense networks do not necessarily imply impoverished support.

The findings in this study imply that individuals *can* function socially and experience community integration despite psychiatric symptomatology. Indeed the indications are that psychiatric symptomatology is not directly implicated in social functioning and social integration, giving some grounds for optimism about the prospects for community care of people with severe long-term mental illnesses.

From the perspectives of residents themselves we get some glimpses of the dimensions of support that facilitated their perceptions of mental well-being, social functioning and social integration. Whilst previous researchers (Pattison et al. 1975; Cohen and Sokolovsky, 1978a; Burt, 1987; Acock and Hurlbert, 1990) have intimated that large networks are conducive to maintaining and improving mental health and social behaviour, this was not the finding here. The nature of support itself was the key factor. Confiding, decision-making and feedback and surveillance were all found to be dimensions of support relevant to residents' perceived mental well-being.

In relation to social functioning household, personal and material support as well as feedback and surveillance were all perceived as implicated. Individual differences in the social functioning of residents were seen very much as a reflection of the contrasting care practices of staff in the separate houses.

The issue of social integration was tackled at different levels. It was self-evident that locational integration or the actual placement of individuals within community settings had taken place for individuals in both housing projects. To a large degree this was the limit of staff expectations at Mountain View.

Environmental integration was considered in terms of the actual building or physical context and the wider community or 'external environment' (Bloor et al. 1988). Both care projects were situated within an environment where usual amenities were available. It was virtually impossible from the outside to distinguish the Greentrees houses from other residential property in the locality. Mountain View was situated alongside or opposite nursing homes for resettled hospital patients. Its size and many interior design features such as its staff room, communal lounge, and lack of individualised furnishings and possessions signalled something akin to a more institutional setting.

Taking another measure of social integration, community activity participation based on Shadish and Bootzin (1984), it was found that passive activity such as watching television or doing nothing were the order of the day, supporting findings elsewhere (Shadish and Bootzin, 1984; Cotterill, 1994). The absence of a coherent policy about employment, day activity and leisure was the principal cause. Residents were not shy to express their boredom and frustration with the present arrangements.

Using network membership as a further measure of social integration, community members including service contacts and social acquaintances formed only a small proportion of residents' networks. Whilst most of the study group were hindered from forming such social alliances by virtue of their psychiatric background, poverty, smoking habits, personal presentation and communication problems, the more interventionist care practices at Greentrees did make some limited impact in expanding opportunities for individuals. By contrast, due to the adopted laissez-faire approach residents of Mountain View did not easily re-acquire the skills necessary for community acceptance and the development of relationships with community members. Thus from the viewpoint of network membership, many individuals' lives were far from integrated with the local community. The danger signals about community care lapsing into segregated care are plain to see.

Residents had a range of insights into forms of social integration which they valued. Locational and environmental dimensions as discussed above were usually implicit but most people latched onto the notion of being able to socialise with ordinary people in the community as the thing they most valued. In most cases there was a close awareness of personal factors (social skills, dependency on medication) or external factors (relative poverty, unemployment, care practices) that mediated a person's ability to become more included in local communities and to develop closer attachments to communities of interest. Some people were quite happy with the way things were but on the whole unfulfilled hopes were more in evidence. Leaving residents to their own devices was a recipe for disappointment and disaster. From the evidence we are convinced that many staff remain unaware that people who are severely mentally ill, behaviourally challenged and dependent on heavy drug regimes can have such incisive and telling insights into factors shaping their social lives.

Policy implications

Set against community care policy expectations (Department of Health, 1989) the findings have a number of policy implications.

Expectations about enabling people to live as normal a life as possible in their own homes or in a homely environment in the community illustrate that this can be fulfilled in terms of the use of ordinary housing. This was very evident in the case of Greentrees which managed to cater for individuals with very disabling long-term psychiatric conditions. The housing was inconspicuous and based in residential neighbourhoods. Despite a small number of early untoward reactions from local residents about the use of ordinary housing for the resettlement of people from long-stay hospital, any fears and anxieties of local residents appeared to give way over time to passive acceptance. The Mountain View house on the other hand presented a large and imposing facade in the main street of a small town. Externally, it looked more like a substantial block of offices or, with so many people venturing in and out, like a hostel of some kind. There is no doubting which of the two models gave the appearance of mirroring ordinary housing designs.

The achievement of 'maximum possible independence' through the provision of the right amount of care and support which the White Paper promotes is rather more difficult to evaluate from the findings of the study. On the one hand the Mountain View project appeared to stress the freedom of individuals to exercise choice and self-determination, something reinforced by adoption of a policy of minimum interference in people's day-to-day lives. This could be construed as stressing the rights of individuals to exercise *autonomy*. *Independence*, on the other hand, was something which had to be learned through making mistakes when community norms were breached, as happened when certain individuals were 'banished' from

public houses or cafés because of inappropriate behaviour. Greentree
more interventionist social and living skills approach (Hayes, 1989)
idea of helping individuals to re-acquire those skills necessary for mor
living. It could be said that the two housing projects were thus
different goals as well as to different means of achieving them. Mor
appear to stand in opposition. The kind of independence stressed in the Gr
houses could only be achieved by interventions which by their nature 'interfered' in people's daily lives and to a degree took away some of their autonomy. On the other hand, the ends that were beginning to be achieved for individuals in personal and social terms suggest that the more structured approach involved was the one to be commended.

The diverging interpretations of the same county policy evident between projects highlights the need for policy aims to be *clearly operationalised.* Continuous assessment of how policy is being operationalised at the local level is vital to guard against possible misinterpretation of original aims and objectives. In the present study, it was found that project philosophy was very much based upon the beliefs of 'who was in charge' which in the case of Mountain View may not have been necessarily synonymous with the intentions of policy makers nor, more importantly, with residents' needs.

Despite the SRV roots of the Mountain View philosophy, the lack of structure in people's daily lives, whilst stressing autonomy, appeared to leave individuals without a purpose for living. Policy guidance perhaps needs to identify more clearly which dimensions of independence, including autonomy, are best achieved through different means, recognising that certain ends may only be achievable through a trade-off with what can present as an over-zealous commitment to particular value-driven means. It seems that under the banner of respecting people's rights to withdraw, there can be dangers in 'minimum intervention' degenerating into 'no intervention'.

There is, however, a fine line to be drawn in deciding what is an acceptable level of involvement in people's lives, particularly for those of retirement age. The family models described in the Greentrees houses sometimes presented as being overly paternal or maternal with residents being treated 'as if' children. To a degree this was also mirrored in the minimisation of risk-taking behaviour adopted by staff. Policies committed to the idea of social rehabilitation of individuals need to recognise that staff will need to take calculated risks about exposing people to the communities in which they live. In this sense there is probably a middle ground to be exploited which falls between the rather polar positions adopted by the two housing projects described.

The findings suggest the need for a coordinated policy thrust which recognised the influence of *structural* as well as *personal* problems in people's lives. At the structural level, the position of relative financial poverty experienced by residents needs to be recognised as presenting a barrier to community participation. This also emerged as an issue in the Care in the Community Demonstration Projects (Knapp et al. 1992). What this suggests is the need for more sympathetic alignment of social security and incomes policy with social care policy so that individuals with long-term mental health problems do not find themselves financially penalised to an extent that is more likely to lead to their exclusion from society. There is also the need for policy to recognise that the lack of tailored employment and educational opportunities for individuals, and a dependence on specialist segregated provision such as day care, can combine to exclude people from fuller participation within the community.

Although individuals were all subject to individual action plan processes, and to formal or informal systems of key workers, it remains the case that there should be a greater emphasis on *targeting* those with the most challenging behaviours. A failure to confront this issue and to find creative solutions to it runs the risk of socially excluding those whose need for help is perhaps greatest. At the more personal level, it is clear that more needs to be done to help people with personal presentation and with communication skills, as both factors were seen to mediate social integration.

Suggestions for further research

Individual outcomes may be regarded as the most important measure of the success or failure of community care policy. Despite this there has been a shortage of studies which specifically address individual outcomes from the user's perspective. If community care is to be truly client-centred, this perspective must become an integral part of service evaluation, with the voice of the consumer heard rather than regarded as a mere product of their illness (Williams, 1995). Methodologically this means that individuals need to be able to tell their own stories and be listened to. The present study has made a modest contribution in this regard but there is much more to be achieved.

Cahill (1994) argues that social policy research needs to be in touch with the *ordinary concerns* of people, especially those who use services. Service users need to be given the opportunity, freedom and help to voice and define their concerns, and in so doing take ownership of the research process as an integral part of being empowered. This raises epistemological, ontological and methodological issues which some consider to be part of new research paradigms in work with people who are disabled or disadvantaged (Rioux and Bach, 1994). Not only would moves in this direction make services and policy-making processes more directly accountable to those who are supposed to benefit from them, it would help to ensure that the research agenda is itself shaped by the expressed concerns of those who have for so long been marginalised in decision-making processes.

At a more mundane level the study has highlighted the limitations of over-dependence on a positivist methodology when seeking to intercept the social lives of people with long-term mental illnesses. Fieldwork suggested that there was a latent, sometimes open, antipathy towards the use of scales and checklists which reminded some individuals of psychiatric interviews. More importantly, there was some evidence to suggest that such dependence may result in data of questionable reliability, especially if produced on days when individuals were 'feeling off'. Ethnography provided a flexible approach which more easily accommodated tailored forms of questioning, and in the end this appeared to generate a different profile of the structural parameters of people's social networks. Were such findings to be generalised they may call into question the assumptions made about the structure and scope of people's networks which have on the whole been based on the findings of studies using quantitative methods (Sokolovsky and Cohen, 1981; Leff et al. 1990; Dunn et al. 1990; Anderson et al. 1993). The effects of different name-eliciting procedures on what we know about the social networks of people with severe mental illnesses seems a subject worthy of further investigation.

A weakness of the present study lies in the realm of the time period in which it was conducted. The experiences reported by residents and staff were conditioned by the relatively recent relocation of residents into community settings. There was not the opportunity to engage in a formal longitudinal study which might reveal different patterns of personal adjustment and community adaptation. Informal contacts with respective housing projects after withdrawal from the field provided only a few glimpses of adaptations, albeit over an extended period of time. Prospective longitudinal network studies in this field would be invaluable in assessing stability and change in the support and social integration of people with severe mental illness in the community.

More studies which mirror the contrastive element of this research would also be useful. As the era of institutionalisation is rapidly coming to an end, individuals are being relocated into various types of physical dwelling as well as differing care structures. The present study has mapped some of the relationships between dimensions of support and types of outcome for service users. More work of this kind is required with the wide range of people presently using community mental health services so that more robust models can be generated as templates for professional practice. Social network and social support theory (Brugha et al. 1993; Cook and Wright, 1995; Eurelings-Bontekoe et al. 1995; Nelson et al. 1992; Uehara 1995) would appear to offer useful frameworks for further model building in this field. Whether there is the commitment to fund 'what is to be done' is now the critical question.

References

Abrahamson, D., Swatton, J. and Wills, W. (1989), 'Do Long-stay Psychiatric Patients Want to Leave Hospital?', *Health Trends,* 21, 17-19.

Acock, A.L. and Hurlbert, J.S. (1990), 'Social Network Analysis: A Structural Perspective for Family Studies', *Journal of Social and Personal Relationships,*7, 245-64.

Alaszewski, A. (1988), 'Institutional Care and the Mentally Handicapped', *Paper Given to the Nursing and Anthropology Association Conference 'Understanding Disability'*, London.

Albrecht, T.L. (1994), 'Epilogue: Social Support and Community: A Historical Account of the Rescue Networks in Denmark', in Burleson, B.R., Albrecht, T.L.and Sarason, I.G. (eds) *Communication of Social Support. Messages, Interactions, Relationships, and Community*, 267-279, London: Sage.

Aldous, J. and Straus, M.A. (1966), 'Social Networks and Conjugal Roles: A Test of Bott's Hypothesis', *Social Forces*, 44, 576-580.

Allen, S. and Watson, A. (1986), 'The Effects of Unemployment: Experience and Response', in Allen, S., Watson, A., Purcell, K. and Wood, S. (eds.), *The Experience of Unemployment*, Ca: Macmillan.

Anderson, J., Dayson, D., Wills, W., Gooch, C., Margolius, O., O'Driscoll, C. and Leff, J. (1993), 'The TAPS Project 13: Clinical and Social Outcomes of Long-Stay Psychiatric Patients After One Year in the Community', *British Journal of Psychiatry,* 162 (suppl. 19), 45-56.

Anderson, M. (1971), 'Family Household and the Industrial Revolution', in Anderson, M. (ed) *Sociology of the Family*, Harmondsworth: Penguin.

Aneshensel, C.S. and Frerichs, R.R. (1982), 'Stress, Support and Depression: A Longitudinal Causal Model', *Journal of Community Psychology*, 10, 363-376.

Aneshensel, C.S. and Stone, J.D. (1982), 'Stress and Depression: A Test of the Buffering Model of Social Support', *Archives of General Psychiatry*, 39, 1392-1396.

Anthony, W.A., Cohen, M.R. and Vitalo, R. (1978), 'The Measurement of Rehabilitation Outcome', *Schizophrenia Bulletin*, 4, 365-383.

Anthony, W.A. and Farkas, M. (1982), 'A Client-Outcome Planning Model for Assessing Psychiatric Rehabilitation Interventions', *Schizophrenia Bulletin*, 8, 13-38.

Anthony, W.A. and Liberman, R.P. (1986), 'The Practice of Psychiatric Rehabilitation. Historical Conceptual and Research Base', *Schizophrenia Bulletin*, 12, 542-559.

Antonovsky, A. (1974), 'Conceptual and Methodological Problems in the Study of Resistance, Resources and Stressful Life Events', in Dohrenwend, B.S. and Dohrenwend, B.P (eds.) , *Stressful Life Events: Their Nature and Effects,* 1974, 245-258, New York: John Wiley.

APA (1980), *Diagnostic and Statistical Manual (DSM-111),* (3rd edition), American Psychiatric Association, Washington D.C.

Audit Commission (1994), *Finding a Place. A Review of Mental Health Services for Adults*, London: HMSO.

Baily, C.A. (1996), *A Guide to Field Research*, Pine Forge Press, London: Sage.

Baker, B.L., Seltzer, G.B. and Seltzer, M.M. (1977), *As Close as Possible,* Boston: Little Brown.

Baker, R. and Hall, J.N. (1983), *Users Manual for Rehabilitation Hall and Baker,* Scotland: Vine.

Barham, P. and Hayward, R. (1991), *From the Mental Patient to the Person,* London and New York: Tavistock/Routledge.

Barnes, J.A. (1954), 'Class and Committees in a Norwegian Island Parish', *Human Relations*, 7, 39-58.

Barrera, M. Jr. (1986), 'Distinctions between Social Support Concepts, Measures and Models', *American Journal of Community Psychology*, 14, 413-45.

Barrera, M. (1978), 'A Method for the Assessment of Social Support Networks in Community Survey Research', *Connections*, 3, 8-15.

Barrera, M. Jr. and Ainlay, S.L. (1983), 'The Structure of Social Support: A Conceptual and Empirical Analysis', *Journal of Community Psychology*, 11, 133-143.

Barry, M.M. and Crosby, C. (1996), 'Quality of Life as an Evaluative Measure in Assessing the Impact of Community Care on People with Long-Term Psychiatric Disorder', *British Journal of Psychiatry*, 168, 210-216.

Barry, M.M. and Crosby, C. (1992), 'Community Mental Health Care: Promoting a Better Quality of Life for Long-Term Clients', *Promotion of Mental Health*, 2.

Barry, M.M., Crosby, C., Bogg, J. and Carter, M.F. (1992), *Brief Report on Client Outcomes at Six Months Post-Discharge,* UCW Bangor: Health Services Research Unit.

Barry, M.M., Crosby, C. and Mitchell, D.A. (1990), 'Paper 3. Quality of Life', in HSRU, *An Interim Report*, UCW Bangor.

Barton, R. (1959), *Institutional Neurosis,* Bristol: John Wright and Sons Ltd.

Bean, P. and Mounser, P. (1993), *Discharged from Mental Hospitals,* Hampshire: Macmillan and MIND.

Becker, H.S. (1963), *Outsiders,* New York: The Free Press.

Becker, H.S., Geer, B., Hughes, E.C. and Strauss, A.L. (1961), *Boys in White*, Chicago: University of Chicago Press.

Beels, C.C. (1981), 'Social Support and Schizophrenia', *Schizophrenia Bulletin,* 7, 58-72.

Belknap, I. (1956), *Human Problems at a State Mental Hospital,* New York: McGraw-Hill.

Bell, C.R. (1968), *Middle Class Families,* London: RKP.

Bellack, A.S. and Meuser, K.T. (1986), 'A Comprehensive Treatment Program for Schizophrenia and Chronic Mental Illness', *Community Mental Health Journal*, 22(3), 175-190.

Bellack, A.S., Morrison, R.L., Wixted, J.T. and Mueser, K.T. (1990), 'An Analysis of Social Competence in Schizophrenia', *British Journal of Psychiatry*, 156, 809-818.

Bennet, D (1978), 'Community Psychiatry', *British Journal of Psychiatry*, 132, 209-20.

Berkowitz, R. (1986), 'Expressed Emotion in Families of Schizophrenic Patients', in Chester, R. and Divall, P. (eds.) , *Mental Health, Illness and Handicap in Marriage,* Rugby: National Marriage Guidance Council.

Blau, Z.S. (1973), *Old Age in a Changing Society*, New York: Franklin Watts.

Bloor, M., McKeganey, N. and Fonkert, D. (1988), *One foot in Eden. A Sociological Study of the Range of Therapeutic Community Practice*, London and New York: Routledge.

Blumer, H. (1969), *Symbolic Interactionism: Perspective and Method,* Englewood Cliffs: N.J. Prentice-Hall, Inc.

Booth, T., Bilson, A. and Fowell, I. (1990), 'Staff Attitudes and Caring Practices in Homes for the Elderly', *British Journal Social Work*, 20, 117-131.

Borchert, J. (1980), *Alley Life in Washington: Family, Community, Religion and Folklife in the City*, 1850-1970.

Bott, E. (1957), Reprint (1971), *Family and Social Networks,* London: Tavistock Publications Limited.

Bowers, B.J. (1987), 'Inter-Generational Caregiving: Adult Caregivers and their Ageing Parents', *Advances in Nursing Science*, 9(2), 20-31.

Bowlby, J. (1980), *Attachment and Loss: Vol. 3, Loss,* New York: Basic books.

Bowlby, J. (1973), *Attachment and Loss: Vol. 2, Separation: Anxiety and Anger,* London: Hogarth Press.

Bowlby, J. (1969), *Attachment and Loss: Vol. 1, Attachment,* London: Hogarth Press.

Brabbins, C., Farell, V. and Cunningham, J. (1995), 'Mental Health Day Care Services; The Patient's Perspective', *Health and Social Care in the Community*, 3, 5, 321-333.

Breier, A.B. and Strauss, J.S. (1984), 'The Role of Social Relationships in the Recovery from Psychotic Disorders', *American Journal of Psychiatry,* 141, 8, 949-955.

Brim, J.A. (1974), 'Social Network Correlates of Avowed Happiness', *Journal of Nervous and Mental Disease,* 58, 432-439.

Brinck, U. (1994), 'Psychiatric Care and Social Support for People with Long-Term Mental Illness in Sweden', *International Journal of Social Psychiatry*, 40, 4, 258-268.

Brindle, D. (1996), 'Move to Plug Care Gap for Mentally Ill', *The Guardian*, 21 February Home Page 5.

Brown, G.W., Bhrolchaim, M.N. and Harris, T. (1975), 'Social Class and Psychiatric Disturbance Among Women in the Urban Population', *Sociology,* 9, 225-254.

Brown, G.W., Bone, M., Dalison, B. and Wing, J.K. (1966), *Schizophrenia and Social Care: A Comparative Follow-up Study of 339 Schizophrenic Patients,* Oxford: Oxford University Press.

Brown, G.W. and Harris, T. (1978), *Social Origins of Depression: A Study of Psychiatric Disorders in Women,* New York: Free Press.

Brown, P. (1985), *The Transfer of Care,* London: Routledge and Kegan Paul.

Brugha, T., Conroy, R., Walsh, N., Delaney, W., O'Hanlon, J., Dondero, E., Daly, L., Hickey, N. and Bourke, G. (1982), 'Social Networks, Attachments and Support in Minor Affective Disorders: A Replication', *British Journal of Psychiatry,* 141, 249-255.

Brugha, T.S., Sturt, E., MacCarthy, B., Potter, J., Wykes, T. and Bebbington, P.E. (1987), 'The Interview Measure of Social Relationships: the Description and Evaluation of a Survey Instrument for Assessing Personal Social Resources', *Social Psychiatry,* 22, 123-128.

Brugha, T.S., Wing, J.K., Brewin, C.R., MacCarthy, B. and Lesage, A. (1993), 'The Relationships of Social Network Deficits in Social Functioning in Long-Term Psychiatric Disorders', *Social Psychiatry and Psychiatric Epidemiology*, 28, 218-224.

Bryman, A. (1989), *Research Methods and Organisation Studies,* Contemporary Social Research Series, 20, London: Unwin Hyman Ltd.

Bryman, A. (1988), *Quantity and Quality in Social Research,* London: Unwin Hyman Ltd.

Buber, M. (1965), *Between Man and Man*, New York: Macmillan.

Buchanan, D., Boddy, D. and McCalman, J. (1988), 'Getting In, Getting On, Getting Out and Getting Back', in Bryman, A. (ed.) *Doing Research in Organizations,* 53-67, London: Routledge.

Bulmer, M. (1987), *The Social Basis of Community Care,* London: Allen and Unwin.

Burgess, R.G. (1984), *In the Field. An Introduction to Field Research,* London: George Allen and Unwin.

Burke, R.J. and Weir, T. (1978), 'Sex Differences in Adolescent Life Stress, Social Support and Well Being', *Journal of Psychology,* 98, 277-288.

Burt, R.S. (1987), 'A Note on Strangers, Friends and Happiness', *Social Networks,* 9, 311-31.

Bury, M. (1992), *Caveat Venditor: Challenges to the Pharmaceutical Industry,* Conference North Wales Regional Meeting Big Business or Successful Science? Psychopharmacology in the Community 27th March 1992.

Butler, R.J. and Rosenthal, G. (1985), *Behaviour and Rehabilitation,* Behavioural Treatment for Long-Stay Patients, (2nd edition).

Cahill, M. (1994), *The New Social Policy,* Oxford: Blackwell.

Caldock, K.J. (1993), *Domiciliary Services for Elderly People: An Analytical critique,* PhD thesis (unpublished), Bangor: University of Wales.

Cambridge, P. and Knapp, M. (1988), *Demonstrating Successful Care in the Community,* Canterbury: PSSRU, University of Kent.

Caplan, G. (1976), 'The Family as Support System' in Caplan, G. and Killiles, M. (eds) *Support Systems and Mutual Help Multidisciplinary Explorations,* New York: Grune and Stratton.

Caplan, G. (1974), *Support Systems and Community Mental Health: Lectures on Concept Development*, New York Behavioural.

Caplan, R., Cobb, S., French, J., Harrison, R. and Pinneau, S. (1980), *Job Demands and Worker Health,* Ann Arbor, MI: Institute for Social Research.

Carling, P.J. (1996), 'Major Mental Illness, Housing and Supports: The Promise of Community Integration', *American Psychologist*, 45, 969-975.

Carstairs, G.M. (1959), *The Social Limits of Eccentricity: an English Study, in Culture and Mental Health: Cross-Cultural Studies*, edited by Opler, M.K., New York: Macmillan.

Carveth, W.B. and Gottlieb, B.H. (1979), 'The Measurement of Social Support and its Relation to Stress', *Canadian Journal of Behavioural Science,* 11, 179-187.

Cassel, J. (1976), 'The Contribution of the Social Environment to Host Resistance', *American Journal of Epidemiology,* 104, 107-123.

Castle, I.M. and Gittus, E. (1957), 'The Distribution of Social Defects in Liverpool', *Sociological Review,* 5, 43-64.

Caton, C. (1984), *Management of Chronic Schizophrenia,* New York: Oxford University Press.

Caudhill, W. (1958), *The Psychiatric Hospital as a Small Society,* Mass.: Harvard University Press.

Chahal, K.K. and Lee-Jones, R. (1993), 'Social Networks of Two Group Homes Five Years On', in preparation quoted in Dayson, D. (1992), 'The TAPS Project 15: The Social Networks of Two Group Settings: A Pilot Study', *Journal of Mental Health,* 1, 99-106.

Cheadle, A.J., Freeman, H. and Korer, J. (1978), 'Chronic Schizophrenic Patients in the Community', *British Journal of Psychiatry,* 132, 221-27.

Cobb, S. (1979), 'Social Support and Health Through the Life Course', in Riley, M.W. (ed.), Ageing from Birth to Death, *Interdisciplinary Perspectives*, 93-106.

Cobb, S. (1976), 'Social Support as a Moderator of Life Stress', *Psychosomatic Medicine,* 38, 300-310.

Cohen, A. P. (1985), *The Symbolic Construction of Community,* London: Routledge (reprinted 1989).

Cohen, B.F. and Anthony W.A. (1984), 'Functional Assessment in Rehabilitation' in Halpern, A.S. and Fuhrer, M.J. (eds) *Functional Assessment in Rehabilitation*, 79-99, Baltimore: Paul Brookes.

Cohen, C.I. and Sokolovsky, J. (1979), 'Clinical Use of Network Analysis for Psychiatric and Aged Populations', *Community Mental Health Journal*, 15, 203-213.

Cohen, C.I. and Sokolovsky, J. (1978a), 'Social Networks and Schizophrenia', *Schizophrenia Bulletin,* 4, 346-360.

Cohen, C.I. and Sokolovsky, J. (1978b), 'Schizophrenia and Social Networks: Ex-patients in the Inner City', *Schizophrenia Bulletin*, 4, 4, 546-560.

Cohen, S., Mermelstein, R., Kamarck, T. and Hoberman, H.N. (1985), 'Measuring the Functional Components of Social Support', in Sarason, I. and Sarason, B. (eds.), *Social Support: Theory, Research and Application,* Dordrecht, The Netherlands: Marinus Nijhoff, 73-94.

Cohen, S. and Wills, T.A. (1985), 'Stress, Social Support and the Buffering Hypothesis', *Psychological Bulletin*, 98, 310-357.

Collins, A.H. and Pancoast, D.L. (1976), *Natural Helping Networks. A Strategy for Prevention,* USA: National Association of Social Workers.

Commerford, M.C. and Reznikoff, M. (1996), 'Relationship of Religion and Perceived Social Support to Self-Esteem and Depression in Nursing Home Residents', *Journal of Psychology*, 130, 1, 35-50.

Cook, J.A. and Wright, E.R. (1995), 'Medical Sociology and the Study of Severe Mental Illness: Reflections on Post Accomplishments and Directions for Future Research', *Journal of Health and Social Behaviour*, (extra issue), 95-114.

Cormack, D.F. (1981), 'Making Use of Unsolicited Research Data', *Journal of Advanced Nursing*, 6, 41-49.

Cotterill, L. (1994), *The Social Integration of People with Schizophrenia,* Aldershot: Avebury.

Craven, P. and Wellman, B. (1973), 'The Network City', *Sociological Inquiry*, 43, 3 and 4, 57-88.

Cresswell, C.M., Kuipers, L. and Powers, M. (1992), 'Social Networks and Support in Long-Term Psychiatric Patients', *Psychological Medicine*, 22, 1019-1026.

Crosby, C. (1990), 'Paper 1. Ward Environments', in HSRU, *An Interim Report*, 5-31, UCW Bangor.

Crosby, C. and Barry, M.M. (1995) (eds), *Community Care: Evaluation of the Provision of Mental Health Services*, Aldershot: Avebury.

Crosby, C., Barry, M.M., Bogg, J. and Carter, M.F. (1992), *Brief Report on the Care Process in Two Community Care Schemes,* UCW Bangor: Health Services Research Unit.

Crosby, C., Barry, M.M. and Geertshuis, S.A. (1995a), 'Psychiatric and Behavioural Outcomes for Clients Twelve Months after Discharge from Hospital', in Crosby, C. and Barry, M.M. (eds), *Community Care Evaluation of the Provision of Mental Health Services*, 87-110, Aldershot, Avebury.

Crosby, C., Barry, M.M., Mitchell, D.A., Horrocks, F. and Littlejohns, C. (1990), *An Interim Report,* UCW Bangor: Health Services Research Unit.

Crosby, C., Carter, M.F. and Barry, M.M. (1995b), 'The Care Process: Care Environments, Care Management and Staff Attitudes', in Crosby, C. and Barry, M.M. (eds.) *Community Care: Evaluation of the Provision of Mental Health Services*, 59-86, Aldershot: Avebury.

Curran, J.P., Marti, P.M. and Corriveau, D.P. (1982), *International Handbook of Behaviour Modification and Therapy,* New York: Plenum Press.

Cutrona, C.E. and Suhr, J.A. (1994), 'Social Support Communication in the Context of Marriage. An Analysis of Couples' Supportive Interactions', in Burleson, B.R., Albrecht, T.L. and Sarason, G.I. (eds) *Communication of Social Support. Messages, Interactions, Relationships, and Community*, 113-135, California: Sage.

d'Abbs, P. (1982), *Social Support Networks: A Critical Review of Models and Findings,* Melbourne: Institute of Family Studies Monograph No 1.

Davey, B. (1994), 'Mental Health and the Evironment', *Care in Place,* 1, 2, June 1994, 188-201.

Dayson, D. (1992), 'The TAPS Project 15: The Social Networks of Two Group Settings: A Pilot Study', *Journal of Mental Health,* 1, 99-106.

Denzin, N.K. (1970), *The Research Act in Sociology: A Theoretical Introduction to Sociological Methods*, London: Butterworths.

Department of Health (1996), *New Mental Health Act Comes into Force*, DoH Information Division Press Release 96/108, 1 April 1996.

Department of Health (1995), *Building Bridges*, HMSO.

Department of Health (1995), *Virginia Bottomley Opens Community Care Charter Conferences*, DoH Information Division Press Release 95/231, 12 May 1995.

Department of Health (1989), *Caring for People. Community Care in the Next Decade and Beyond*, cm 849, London: HMSO.

Dilks, S.L.E. and Shattock, L. (1996), 'Does Community Residence Mean More Community Contact for People with Severe, Long-Term Psychiatric Disabilities?' *British Journal of Clinical Psychology*, 35, 183-192.

Dincin, J. (1975), 'Psychiatric Rehabilitation', *Schizophrenia Bulletin,* 13, 131-147.

Dinitz, S., Lefton, M. and Angrist, S. (1967), 'Psychiatric and Social Attributes as Predictors of Case Outcome in Mental Hospitalization' in Scheff, T.J. (ed.) *Mental Illness and Social Processes*, New York: Harper and Row.

Douglas, J.D. (1985), *Creative Interviewing*, Beverley Hills, CA: Sage.

Drass, K.A. (1980), 'The Analysis of Qualitative Data: A Computer Program', *Urban Life,* 9, 322-353.

Dufåker, M. (1994), 'Discharge Procedures for Mentally Ill People. The Perspective of Former Psychiatric Patients on Their Professioal Social Network', *Scand.J.Soc.Welfare*, 3, 7-13

Dumont, M.P. (1967), 'Tavern Culture: The Sustenance of Homeless Men', *American Journal of Orthopsychiatry*, 37, 938-945.

Dunham, H.W. and Weinberg, S.K. (1960), *The Culture of the State Mental Hospital,* Detroit: Wayne State University Press.
Dunn, M., O'Driscoll, C., Dayson, D., Wills, W. and Leff, J. (1990), 'The TAPS Project 4: An Observational Study of the Social Life of Long-Stay Patients', *British Journal of Psychiatry,* 157, 842-848.
Durkheim, E. (1952), *Suicide: A Study in Sociology,* London: Routledge and Kegan Paul (first published 1897).
Dworkin, R. (1992), *Researching Persons with a Mental Illness*, CA: Sage.
Edwards, A. and Talbot, R. (1994), *The Hard-Pressed Researcher*, A Research Handbook for the Caring Professions, Essex: Longman.
Eggert, C., Granger, V., Morris, R. and Pendleton, S. (1977), 'Caring for the Patient with a Long-term Disability', *Geriatrics*, 32, 107.
Eisemann, M. and Perris, C. (1985), 'Social Support In Non-Psychotic Psychiatric Outpatients' in *Psychiatry: The State of the Art Vol 7 Epidemiology and Community Psychiatry*, 135-139.
Ekeh, P.P. (1974), *Social Exchange Theory: The Two Traditions,* Cambridge, MA: Harvard University Press.
Ell, K. (1996), 'Social Networks, Social Support and Coping with Serious Illness: The Family Connection', *Social Science and Medicine*, 42, 2, 173-183.
Ellsworth, R.B., Foster, L., Childers, B., Arthur, G. and Krocker, D. (1968), 'Hospital and Community Adjustment as Perceived by Psychiatric Patients, their Families and Staff', *Journal of Consulting and Clinical Psychology* (monograph supplement) 32, 1-41.
Englehardt, P.M. and Rosen, B. (1976), 'Implications of Drug Treatment for the Social Rehabilitation of Schizophrenic Patients', *Schizophrenic Bulletin,* 2, 454-462.
Estroff, S.E. (1995), 'Brokenhearted Lifetimes: Ethnography, Subjectivity and Psychosocial Rehabilitation', *International Journal of Mental Health*, 24, 1, 82-92.
Estroff, S.E. (1985), *Making it Crazy. An Ethnography of Psychiatric Clients in an American Community,* California: University of California Press.
Eurelings-Bontekoe, E.H.M., Diekstra, R.F.W. and Verschuur, M. (1995), 'Psychological Distress, Social Support and Social Support Seeking: A Prospective Study Among Primary Mental Health Care Patients', *Social Science and Medicine,* 40, 8, 1083-1089.
Faber, S. (1993), *Madness, Heresy and the Rumor of Angels: The Revolt Against the Mental Health System*, Chicago: Open Court.
Fagin, L. and Little, M. (1984), *The Forsaken Families*, London: Fontana.
Fetterman, D.M. (1989), *Ethnography. Step by Step*, Applied Social Research Methods Series Volume 17, London: Sage Publications.
Field, P.A. and Morse, J.M. (1991), *Nursing Research: The Application of Qualitative Approaches,* London: Chapman and Hall.
Fielding, N. (1993), 'Ethnography', in Gilbert, N. (ed.), *Researching Social Life*, 9, 154-171, London: Sage.

Filstead, W.J. (1979), 'Qualitative Methods: a needed perspective in evaluation research', in Cook, T.D. and Reichardt, C.S. (eds) , *Qualitative and Quantitative Methods in Evaluation Research,* Beverly Hills, Cal.: Sage, 33-48.

Fischer, C.S. (1977), 'Network Analysis and Urban Studies', in Fischer C.S. et al., *Networks and Places: Social Relations in the Urban Setting*, 19-37, New York, Free Press.

Fischer, C.S. (1976), *The Urban Experience*, Chicago: Harcourt Brace Jovanovich.

Fischer, C.S. and Phillips, S.L. (1982), 'Who is Alone? Social Characteristics of People With Small Networks', in Peplau, L.A. and Perlman, D. (eds), *Loneliness, A Source of Current Theory, Research and Therapy,* New York: John Wiley, 21-39.

Florian, V., Mikulincer, M. and Bucholtz, I. (1995), 'Effects of Adult Attachment Style on the Perception and Search for Social Support', *Journal of Psychology*, 129 (6), 665-676.

Flynn, R.J. and Nitsche, K.E. (eds), (1980), *Normalisation, Social Integration and Community Services,* Baltimore: University Park Press.

Forrester-Jones, R.V.E. (1995), *One Step to Freedom? An Applied Social Network and Ethnographic Study of People with Long-Term Mental Health Problems Re-settled from Hospital to the Community*, PhD Thesis, University of Wales, Bangor.

Forrester-Jones, R. and Grant, G. (1995), 'Social Networks and Lives of People with Long-term Mental Health Problems' in Crosby, C. and Barry, M.M. (eds), *Community Care: Evaluation of The Provision of Mental Health Services,* 111-136 Aldershot: Avebury.

Foucault, M. (1961), 'Folie et Deraison:histoire de la folie al'age classique', trans. Howard, R. (1972) as *Madness and Civilization*, London: Tavistock.

Freeman, H.E. and Simmons, O.G. (1963), *The Mental Patient Comes Home,* New York: John Wiley and Sons.

Froland, C., Brodsky, G., Olson, M. et al (1979), 'Social Support and Social Adjustment: Implications for Mental Health Professionals', *Community Mental Health Journal*, 15, 82-92.

Garety, P. (1988), 'Housing', in Lavender, A. and F. Holloway, F. (eds), *Community Care in Practice: Services for the Continuing Care Client,* Chichester: Wiley.

Gassaway, B.M. and Elder, W.L. (1981), 'Toward De-stigmatizing Computers for Qualitative Sociology: A Methodological Essay. Paper Presented at the Annual Meeting of the Midwest Sociological Society', in Seidel, J.V. and Clark, J.A. (1984), The Ethnograph: A Computer Program for the Analysis of Qualitative Data, *Qualitative Sociology,* 711-721.

Geertz, C. (1973), *'The Interpretation of Cultures: Selected Essays'*, New York: Basic Books.

Geller, J.L. and Harris, M. (1994), *Women of the Asylum: Voices from Behind the Walls*, 1840-1945, New York: Doubleday.

Gerstel, N., Riessman, C.K. and Rosenfield, S. (1985), *Explaining the Symptomatology of Separated and Divorced Women and Men: the Role of Material Conditions and Social Networks.*

Giddens, A. (1992), *The Transformation of Intimacy: Love, Sexuality and Eroticism in Modern Societies,* Cambridge: Polity Press.

Giddens, A. (1989) (2nd edition 1994), *Sociology,* Cambridge: Polity Press.

Giggs, J.A. (1986), 'The distribution of Schizophrenics in Nottingham', *Trans. Int. Brit. Geographers,* 59, 55-76.

Glaser, B.G. and Strauss, A.L. (1967), *The Discovery of Grounded Theory: Strategies for Qualitative Research,* Chicago: Aldine.

Glynn, S. and Mueser, K.T. (1986), 'Social Learning for Chronic Mental Patients', *Schizophrenia Bulletin,* 12, 648-668.

Goering, P., Durbin, J., Foster, R., Boyles, S., Babiak, T. and Lancee, B. (1992), 'Social Networks of Residents in Supportive Housing', *Community Mental Health Journal,* 28(3), 199-214.

Goffman, E. (1961), *Asylums: Essays on the Social Situation of Mental Patients and Other Inmates,* Harmondsworth: Penguin.

Goldstron, I.D. and Manderscheid, R.W. (1982), 'The Chronically Mentally Ill in Community Support Systems', *Community Support Service Journal,* 2, 4-9.

Gottlieb, B.H. (1985), 'Assessing and Strengthening the Impact of Social Support on Mental Health', *Social Work,* July-August, 293-300.

Gottlieb, B.H. (1983), *Social Support Strategies: Guidelines for Mental Health Practice,* Beverly Hills: Sage.

Gottlieb, B.H. (1978), 'The Development and Application of a Classification Scheme of Informal Helping Behaviours', *Canadian Journal of Behavioural Science,* 10, 105-115.

Gouldner, A.W. (1960), 'The Norm of Reciprocity: A Preliminary Statement', *American Sociological Review,* 25, 161-178.

Granovetter, M. (1982), 'The Strength and Weak Ties. A Network Theory Revisited', in Marsden, P.V. and Lin, N. (eds.), *Social Structure and Network Analysis,* 105-130.

Grant, G. (1993), 'Support Networks and Transitions over Two Years Amongst Adults with a Mental Handicap', *Mental Handicap Research,* 6, 36-55.

Grant, G. and McGrath, M. (1990), 'Need for Respite Care Services Among Caregivers of Persons with Mental Retardation', *American Journal on Mental Retardation,* 94, 638-648.

Grant, G. and Wenger, G.C. (1993), 'Dynamics of Support Networks: Differences and Similarities between Vulnerable Groups', *The Irish Journal of Psychology,* 14, 1, 79-98.

Greenblatt, M., Becerra, R.M. and Serafetinides, E.A. (1982), 'Social Networks and Mental Health: An Overview', *The American Journal of Psychiatry,* 139, 8, 977-984.

Gumperz, J. (1981), 'Conversational Inference and Classroom Learning', in Green, J.L. and Wallat, C. (eds), *Ethnography and Language in Educational Settings.* Norwood, N.J.: Ablex.

Hadley, R. and Webb, A. (1974), *Loneliness, Social Isolation and Old People,* London: Age Concern.

Hall, J.N., Baker, R.D. and Hutchinson, K. (1977), 'A Controlled Evaluation of Token Economy Procedures with Chronic Psychiatric Patients', *Behaviour Research and Therapy*, 15, 261-83.

Halpern, A.S. and Fuhrer, M.J. (1984) (eds), *Functional Assessment in Rehabilitation,* Baltimore: Paul Brookes.

Ham, C. (1992), *Health Policy in Britian: The Politics and Organisation of the National Health Service* (3rd edition), Basingstoke: Macmillan.

Hammer, M. (1981), 'Social Supports, Social Networks and Schizophrenia', *Schizophrenia Bulletin*, 7, 45-57.

Hammer, M., Makiesky-Barrow, S. and Gutwirth, L. (1978), 'Social Networks and Schizophrenia', *Schizophrenia Bulletin,* 4, 522-545.

Hammersley, M. and Atkinson, P. (1983), *Ethnography: Principles in Practice*, London: Tavistock.

Hampson, R., Judge, K. and Renshaw, J. (1984), 'Care in the Community Project Material', Canterbury: PSSRU, University of Kent, DHSS (1983), Circular HC(83)6, in Raynes N., *Annotated Directory of Measures of Environmental Quality for Use in Residential Services for People with a Mental Handicap,* 54-55, University of Manchester: Department of Social Policy and Social Work.

Handy, C. (1993), *Understanding Organizations*, London: Penguin Books.

Hare, E.H. (1956), Family Settings and the Distribution of Schizophrenia, *Journal of Mental Science,* 102, 753.

Harris, C.C. (1969), *The Family*, London: Allen and Unwin.

Hart, E. and Bond, M. (1995), *Action Research for Health and Social Care: A Guide to Practice*, Buckingham: Open University Press.

Hayes, R.(1989), 'Occupational Therapy in the Treatment of Schizophrenia', *Occupational Therapy in Mental Health*, 9, 3.

Healy, D. (1991), 'The Ethics of Psychopharmacology', *Choices*, 4.

Henderson, A.S. (1985), 'Social Relationships and the Onset of Depressive Disorders: The Limitations of Social Variables for Aetiological Research', *Psychiatry: The State of the Art of Epidemiology and Community Psychiatry,* 7, 45-51.

Henderson, S. (1977), 'The Social Network, Support and Neurosis: The Function of Attachment in Adult Life', *British Journal of Psychiatry,* 131, 185-91.

Henderson, S., Byrne, D.G., Duncan-Jones, P., Scott, R. and Adcock, S. (1980), 'Social Relationships, Adversity and Neurosis: A Study of Associations in a General Population Sample', *British Journal of Psychiatry*, 136, 574-583.

Henderson, S., Duncan-Jones, P., Byrne, D.G. and Scott, R. (1980), 'Measuring Social relationships: The Interview Schedule for Social Interaction', *Psychological Medicine*, 10, 723-734.

Hirsch, B.J. (1979), 'Psychological Dimensions of Social Networks: A Multimethod Analysis', *American Journal of Community Psychology,* 7, 263-277.
HMSO (1995), *The Mental Health (Patients in the Community) Act*, c.52, London: HMSO.
HMSO (1991), *Standard Occupational Classification Volume 3. A Publication of the Government Statistical Service,* Office of Population Censuses and Surveys, London: HMSO.
HMSO (1990), *National Health Service and Community Care Act*, London HMSO.
Hockey, J. and James, A. (1988), 'Growing Up and Growing Old: Metaphors of Ageing in Contemporary Britain', ASA Conference Papers, London, in Perring, C. (1993), *The Experience of Psychiatric Hospital Closure*, Hants: Avebury.
Holahan, C.J. and Moos, R.H. (1981), 'Social Support and Psychological Distress: A Longitudinal Analysis', *Journal of Abnormal Psychology*, 90, 365-370.
Holloway, F. and Faulkner, A. (1994), 'Psychiatric Hospital Reprovision and the Long Stay Patient: Clinical Outcome and the User Perspective', *Journal of Mental Health,* 3, 241-248.
Holmes-Eber, P. and Riger, S. (1990), 'Hospitalization and the Composition of Mental Patients' Social Networks', *Schizophrenia Bulletin,* 16, 157-164.
Holstein, J.A. and Gubrium, J.F. (1995), *The Active Interview*, Qualitative Research Methods Series 37, A Sage University paper.
Horwitz, A. (1977), 'Social Networks and Pathways to Psychiatric Treatment', *Social Forces*, 56, 81-105.
Hoult, J., Reynolds, R., Charbonneau-Powis, M., Coles, P. and Briggs, J. (1981), 'Psychiatric Hospital Versus Community Treatment: the Results of a Randomized Trial', *Australia and New Zealand Journal of Psychiatry,* 17, 160-167.
House, J.S. (1981), *Work Stress and Social Support,* M.A.: Addison-Wesley.
House, J.S., Umberson, D. and Landis, K.R. (1988), 'Structures and Processes of Social Support', *Annual Review of Sociology*, 14, 293-318.
Howe, G. (1995) *Working with Schizophrenia: A Needs Based Approach*, London: Jessica Kingsley.
Huxley, P., Hagan, T., Hennelly, R. and Hunt, J. (1990), *Effective Community Mental Health Services*, Aldershot: Avebury.
Irving, H.W. (1975), 'Distance, Intensity, Kinship - Key Dimensions of Social Interaction', *Sociology and Social Research*, 60, 70-86.
Jenner, F.A., Monteiro, A.C.D., Zagalo-Cardoso, J.A. and Cunha-Oliveira, J.A. (1993), *Schizophrenia: A Disease or a Way of Being?* Sheffield: Academic Press.
Jick, T.D. (1979), 'Mixing Qualitative and Quantitative methods: Triangulation in Action', *Administrative Science Quarterly*, 24, 602-611.
Johnson, C.L. (1983), 'Dyadic Family Relations and Social Support', *The Gerontologist,* 23, 4, 1983.
Johnstone, E.C., Owens, D.C.G., Gold, A., Crow, T.J. and Macmillan, J.F. (1984), 'Schizophrenic Patients Discharged From Hospital - a Follow-up Study', *British Journal of Psychiatry*, 149, 537-40.

Johnstone, L. (1993), 'Family Management in "Schizophrenia": Its Assumptions and Contradictions', *Journal of Mental Health*, 2, 255-69.

Jones, K. (1995), Foreward to *Working with Schizophrenia: A Needs Based Approach*, Howe, G., London: Jessica Kingsley.

Jones, K. (1988), *Experience in Mental Health Community Care and Social Policy*, London: Sage.

Jones, K., Robinson, M. and Golightly, M. (1986), 'Long-term Psychiatric Patients in the Community', *British Journal of Psychiatry*, 149, 537-40.

Joseph, M. (1990), *Sociology for Everyone*, Cambridge: Polity Press, (2nd edition).

Kahn, R.L. and Antonucci, T.C. (1980), 'Convoys Across the Life Course: Attachment, Roles and Social Support', in Baltes, P.B. and Brim, O.G. (eds) *Life Span Development and Behaviour*, 3, Boston: Lexington Press.

Kaplan, B.H., Cassel, J.C. and Gore, S. (1977), 'Social Support and Health', *Medical Care*, 15(5), Supplement: 47-58.

Katz, M.M. and Lyerly, S.B. (1963), 'Methods for Measuring Adjustment and Social Behaviour in the Community. I: Rationale, Description, Discriminative Validity, and Scale Development', *Psychol Rep.*, 13, 503-535.

Kelvin, P. and Jarrett, J.E. (1985), *Unemployment. Its Social Psychological Effects*, Cambridge: CUP.

Kempen, G.I.J.M. and Eijk, L.M. van (1995), 'The Psychometric Properties of the SSL 1201, A Short Scale for Measuring Social Support in the Elderly', *Social Indicators Research*, 35, 303-312.

Kesey, K. (1962), *One Flew Over the Cuckoo's Nest*, New York: The New American Library.

Khan, V.S. (1979), 'Work and Network. South Asian Woman in South London', *Social Science Research Council*, 114-133, London: MacMillan Press.

Kinard, E.M. (1995), 'Perceived Social Support and Competence in Abused Children: A Longitudinal Perspective', *Journal of Family Violence*, 10, 1, 73-98.

King, R.D., Raynes, N.V. and Tizard, J. (1971), *Patterns of Residential Care*, London: Routledge and Kegan Paul.

Knapp, M., Cambridge, C.T., Beecham, J., Allen, C. and Darton, R. (1994), 'Residential Care as an Alternative to Long-Stay Hospital: A Cost-Effectiveness Evaluation of Two Pilot Projects', *International Journal of Geriatric Psychiatry*, 9, 297-304.

Knapp, M.R.J., Cambridge, P., Thomason, C., Beecham, J.K., Allen, C. and Darton, R.A. (1992), *Care in the Community: Challenge and Demonstration*, Aldershot: Ashgate.

Knapp, M., Cambridge, P., Thomason, C., Beecham, J.K. and Darton, R.A. (1990), *Care in the Community: Lessons from the Demonstration Programme*, Canterbury: University of Kent, PSSRU.

Korman, N. and Glennerster, H. (1990), *Hospital Closure*, Milton Keynes: Open University Press.

Krawiecka, M., Goldberg, D. and Vaughn, M. (1977), 'A Standardized Psychiatric Assessment Scale for Rating Chronic Psychotic Patients', *Acta Psychiatrica Scandinavica*, 55, 299-308.

Kreisman, D.E. and Joy, V.D. (1974), 'Family Response to the Mental Illness of a Relative: A Review of the Literature', *Schizophrenia Bulletin*, 1, 34-57.

Krippendorf, K. (1980), *Content Analysis. An Introduction to its Methodology,* London: Sage.

Kropotkin, P. (1914), *Mutual Aid*, Boston: Extending Horizon Books.

Lamb, R.H. (1984), 'Alternatives to Hospitals', in Talbott, J.A. (ed.) *The Chronic Mental Patient*, London: Grune Stratton.

Langan, M. (1991), 'Community Care in the 1990s: the Community Care White Paper "Caring for People"', *Critical Social Policy*, 29, 58-70.

Laslett, P. (ed.) (1972), *Household and Family in Past Time,* Cambridge: Cambridge University Press.

Laurance, J. (1986), 'Unemployment: Health Hazards', *New Society,* 21 March.

Lea, J. and Young, J. (1984), *What is to be Done About Law and Order?* Harmondsworth: Penguin.

Leavy, R.L. (1983), 'Social Support and Psychological Disorder: A Review', *Journal of Community Psychology,* 11, 3-21.

Lebowitz, B.D. (1980), 'Old Age and Family Functioning', *Journal of Gerontological Social Work,* 1, 111-118.

Lee, R.M. and Renzetti, C.M. (1990), 'The Problems of Researching Sensitive Topics: An Overview and Introduction', *American Behavioural Scientist*, 33, 510-38.

Leff, J., O'Driscoll, C., Dayson, D., Wills, W. and Anderson, J. (1990), 'The TAPS Project. 5: The Structure of Social Network Data obtained from Long-Stay Patients', *British Journal of Psychiatry*, 57, 848-852.

Lefley, H.P. (1996), *Family Caregiving in Mental Illness*. Family Caregiver Applications Series, 7, London: Sage.

Lehman, S. (1980), 'The Social Ecology of Natural Supports', in Jeger, A. and Slotnick, R.W. (eds) , *Community Mental Health: A Behaviour-Ecological Perspective*, New York: Plenum Press, 319-331.

Lehr, U. (1981), 'Consistency and Change in Family Role Activity and Satisfaction in Old Age', paper presented at International Congress of Gerontology, Hamburg, referenced in Wenger, G.C. (1992), *Help in Old Age - Facing Up To Change. A Longitudinal Network Study,* Liverpool: Liverpool University Press.

Lemert, E. (1951), *Social Pathology,* New York: McGraw-Hill.

Lewis, A. and Trieman, N. (1995), 'The TAPS Project 29: Residential Care Provision in North London: A Representative Sample of Ten Facilities for Mentally Ill People', *International Journal of Social Psychiatry*, 42, 4, 257-267.

Lieberman, M.A. (1982), 'The Effects of Social Supports in Response to Stress', in Goldberger, L. and Breznitz, S. (eds), *Handbook of Stress,* New York: Free Press.

Lin, N. and Dean, A. (1985), 'Social Support in the Etiology of Depression. A Panel Study', in *Psychiatry: The State of the Art*, 7, 123-128.

Lin, N., Simeone, R.S., Ensel, W.M. and Kuo, W. (1979), 'Social Support, Stressful Life Events and Illness', *Journal of Health and Social Behaviour*, 20, 108-119.
Lipton, F., Cohen, C., Fischer, E. and Katz, S. (1981), 'Schizophrenia: A Network Crisis', *Schizophrenia Bulletin*, 7, 90-100.
Litwak, E. and Szelenyi, J. (1969), 'Primary Group Structures and their Functions: Kin, Neighbours and Friends', *American Sociological Review*, 34, 4, 468-481.
Lofland, J. and Lofland, L.H. (1984), *Analyzing Social Settings: A Guide to Qualitative Observation and Analysis*, Belmont, California: Wadsworth (2nd edition).
Lowenthal, M.F. and Haven, C. (1968), 'Interaction and Adaptation: Intimacy as a Critical Variable', *American Sociological Review*, 33, 20-30.
Lutz, F.W. (1981), 'Ethnography - The Holistic Approach to Understanding Schooling', in Green, J.L. and Wallat, C. (eds), *Ethnography and Language in Educational Settings*, Norwood, N.J.: Ablex.
Malin, N. (1987) (ed.) , *Reassessing Community Care*, London: Croom Helm.
Malinowski, B. (1935), *Coral Gardens and Their Magic: A Study of the Methods of Tilling the Soil and of Agricultural Rites in the Trobriand Islands*, London: Allen and Unwin.
Marks, I. (1992), 'Innovations in Mental Health Care Delivery', *British Journal of Psychiatry*, 160,589-97.
Martin, J.P. (1984), *Hospitals in Trouble*, Oxford: Blackwell.
McCourt Perring, C. (1993), *The Experience of Psychiatric Hospital Closure. An Anthropological Study*, Aldershot: Avebury.
McFarlane, A.H., Norman, G.R., Streiner, D.L. and Roy, R.G. (1984), 'Characteristics and Correlates of Effective and Ineffective Social Supports', *Journal of Psychosomatic Research*, 28, 6, 501-510.
McGill, P. (1987), 'Sunset in the East', *Observer*, 2 August.
McGrath, M. (1991), *Multidisciplinary Teamwork*, Aldershot: Avebury.
McKinley, J. (1973), 'Social Networks, Lay Consultation and Help-Seeking Behaviour', *Social Forces*, 51, 275-92.
McNeice, F. (1996), *Undercover Britain: Shabby Treatment*, Channel 4, 11 April..
Mead, G. H. (1934), *Mind, Self and Society*, Chicago: University of Chicago Press.
Meise, U. and Fleischhacker, W.W. (1996), 'Perspectives on Treatment Needs in Schizophrenia', *British Journal of Psychiatry*, 168, (suppl. 29), 9-16.
Melzer, D., Hale, A.S., Malik, S.J., Hogman, G.A. and Wood, S. (1991), 'Community Care for Patients with Schizophrenia One Year after Hospital Discharge', *British Medical Journal*, 303, 26th October, 1023-6.
Meltzer, E., Kemp, P. and Smith, B. (1994), 'Social Networks in a Cluster of Three Group Homes for the Mentally Ill', *Journal of Mental Health*, 3, 263-270.
Mental Health Social Work Research and Staff Development Unit (1993), *Certificate in Mental Health Care*, England: University of Manchester, Department of Psychiatry.
Miller, K. and Ray, E.B. (1994), 'Beyond the Ties that Bind: Exploring the "Meaning" of Supportive Messages and Relationships, in Burleson, B.R.,

Albrecht, T.L. and Sarason, I.G. (eds), *Communication of Social Support, Messages, Interactions, Relationships, and Community*, 215-228.

Mitchell, D.A., Crosby, C. and Barry, M.M. (1995), 'Methodology and Cohort Description', in Crosby, C. and Barry, M.B. (eds), *Community Care: Evaluation of the Provision of Mental Health Services,* Aldershot: Avebury.

Mitchell, D.A., Crosby, C., Barry, M.M., Horrocks, F.A. and Littlejohns, C.S. (1990), 'Paper 2, Cohort Description: Demographic, Psychiatric and Behavioural Characteristics', in HSRU (October 1990), *An Interim Report,* UCW Bangor.

Mitchell, E.S. (1986), 'Multiple Triangulation: a Methodology for Nursing Science', *Advances in Nursing Science*, 8, 3, 18-37.

Mitchell, J.C.(ed.) (1969), *Social Networks in Urban Situations,* Manchester University Press.

Moon, G. (1988), 'Is there One Round Here? Investigation Reaction To Small-scale Mental Health Hostel Provision in Portsmouth, England' in Smith, C.G. and Giggs, J.A. (eds), *Location and Stigma,* London: Unwin Hyman, 203-23.

Morris, J. (1993), '"Us" and "Them"? Feminist Research and Community Care', in Bornat, J., Pereira, C., Pilgrim, D. and Williams, F., *Community Care - a Reader,* 156-166, London: The Macmillan Press.

Murrell, S.A., Chipley, Q.T. and Norris, F.H. (1992), 'Functional Versus Structural Social Support, Desirable Events, and Positive Affect in Older Adults', *Psychology and Aging*, 7, 4, 562-570.

Nadel, S.F. (1957), *The Theory of Social Structure,* London: Cohen and West.

Nelson, G., Hall, G.B., Squire, D. and Walsh-Bowers, R.T. (1992), 'Social Network Transactions of Psychiatric Patients', *Social Science and Medicine*, 34, 4, 433-445.

Neuman, W.L. (1991), *Social Research Methods: Qualitative and Quantitative Approaches*, Boston: Allyn and Bacon.

Newby, H. (1977), *The Deferential Worker*, London: Allen Lane.

Nguyen, S.D. and Cebulski, L. (1987), 'Planning Psychiatric Treatment and Rehabilitation For the Long-Term Patient', *Psychiatr. J. Univ. Ottawa*, 12, 1, 9-13.

Nirje, B. (1969), 'The Normalisation Principle and its Human Management Implications', in Kugel, R. and Wolfensberger, W. (eds.), *Changing Patterns in Residential Services for the Mentally Retarded*, 179-195, Washington: DC Government Printing Office.

Nolan, M. and Grant, G. (1992), *Regular Respite. An Evaluation of a Hospital Rota Bed Scheme for Elderly People,* Age Concern Institute of Gerontology Research Paper No. 6., London: Age Concern.

Nolan, M., Keady, J. and Grant, G. (1995), 'Developing a Typology of Family Care: Implications for Users and Other Service Providers', *Journal of Advanced Nursing*, 21, 256-265.

Oakley, A. (1974), *The Sociology of Housework,* Oxford: Martin Robertson.

O'Brien, J. (1994), 'Down Stairs That Are Never Your Own: Supporting People with Developmental Disabilities in Their Own Homes', *Mental Retardation*, 32, 1-6.

O'Brien, J. and Lyle, C. (1989), *Framework for Accomplishments,* Georgia: Responsive Systems Associates.

Orr, E., Thein, R.D. and Aronson, E. (1995), 'Orthopeadic Disability, Conformity and Social Support', *Journal of Psychology*, 129 (2), 203-219.

Parsons, T. (1951), *The Social System,* Glencoe Ill: The Free Press.

Pattison, E.M. (1977), 'Theoretical Empirical Base for Social Systems Therapy', in Foulkes, E., Wintrop, R., Westermeyer, J. and Favazza, A. (eds), *Current Perspectives in Cultural Psychiatry,* 217-253, New York: Spectrum.

Pattison, E.M., DeFrancisco, D., Wood, P., Frazier, H. and Crowder, J. (1975), 'A Psychosocial Kinship Model for Family Therapy', *American Journal of Psychiatry,* 132, 1246-1251.

Pattison, E.M., Llasmas, R. and Hurd, G. (1979), 'Social Network Mediation of Anxiety', *Psychiatric Annals,* 9, 56-67.

Patton, M.Q. (1990), *Qualitative Evaluation and Research Methods,* London: Sage (2nd edition).

Paykel, E.S., Emms, E.M., Fletcher, J. and Rassaby, E.S. (1980), 'Life Events and Social Support in Puerperal Depressions', *British Journal of Psychiatry,* 136, 339-346.

Pearlin, L. (1992), 'Structure and Meaning in Medical Sociology', *Journal of Health and Social Behaviour*, 33, 1-9.

Pearlin, L., Lieberman, M.A., Menaghan, E.G. and Mullan, J.T. (1981), 'The Stress Process', *Journal of Health and Social Behaviour*, 22, 337-356.

Perkins, R.E., Hollyman, J.A., Boardman, C.J., Humphreys-Hunt, B., Reeves, C. and Weizemann, E. (1992), 'From Long-Stay Patient to Sloane Ranger: Outcome of Resettlement of 15 Old-Long-Stay Psychiatric Patients in Warden Supervised Accommodation for the Elderly', *Journal of Mental Health,* 1, 149-162.

Perring, C. (1992), 'The Experience and Perspectives of Patients and Care Staff of the Transition from Hospital to Community-Based Care', in Ramon, S., *Psychiatric Hospital Closure. Myth and Realities,* 122-168, London: Chapman and Hall.

Pickard, L. (1992), 'An Interview with Clients in Residential Mental Health Services', in Pickard, L., Proudfoot, R., Wolfson, D., Clifford, P., Holloway F. and Lindesay, J. (eds), *Evaluating the Closure of Cane Hill Hospital. Final Report of the Cane Hill Research Team,* London: RDP.

Pilling, S. (1991), *Rehabilitation and Community Care,* London and New York: Routledge.

Pinneau, S.R. (1975), 'Effects of Social Support On Psychological and Physiological Strains', unpublished doctoral dissertation, The University of Michigan, referenced in Kahn, R.L. and Antonucci, T.C. (1980), 'Convoys Over The Life Course: Attachment, Roles and Social Support', *Life-Span Development and Behaviour*, 3.

Plas, J., Hoover-Dempsey, K. and Wallston, B. (1985), 'A Conceptualisation of Professional Women's Interpersonal Fields: Social Support, Reference Groups and Persons-To-Be-Reckoned-With', in Sarason, I.G. and Sarason, B.R. (eds.), *Social Support: Theory, Research and Applications*, 187-204, Boston: Martinus Nijhoff.

Pratt, M.W., Luszcz, M.A. and Brown, M.E. (1980), 'Measuring Dimensions of the Quality of Care in Small Community Residences', *American Journal of Mental Deficiency*, 85, 2, 188-194.

Presley, A.S., Grulb, A.B. and Semple, D. (1982), 'Predictors of Successful Rehabilitation in Long-stay Patients', *Acta Psychiatrica Scandinavica,* , 66, 83-88.

Prior, L. (1993), *The Social Organization of Mental Illness,* London: Sage Publications.

Powell, J. E. (1961), 'Speech by the Minister of Health, the Rt. Hon. Enoch Powell', report of the Annual Conference of the National Association for Mental Health, London: *Report of the Annual Conference of the NAMH.*

Qureshi, H., Challis, D. and Davies, B. (1989), *Helpers in Case-Managed Community Care,* Aldershot: Gower.

Qureshi, H. and Walker, A. (1989), *The Caring Relationship. Elderly People and Their Families,* London: Macmillan.

Race, D. (1987), 'Normalisation, Theory and Practice', in Malin, N. (ed.), *Reassessing Community Care*, London: Croom Helm.

Ragin, A.B., Pogue-Geile, M. and Otmanns, T.F. (1989), 'Poverty of Speech in Schizophrenia and Depression During In-patient and Post-hospital Periods', *British Journal of Psychiatry,* 154, 52-57.

Ramon, S. (1991) (ed.), *Beyond Community Care: Normalisation and Integration Work*, London: MIND.

Reda, S. (1994), 'A Study of Twenty Psychiatric Patients Moved from Hospital to Community: Baseline, Six Months and One Year Follow Up', *Journal of Mental Health,* 3, 249-255.

Reid, I. (1989), *Social Class Differences in Britain: Life-Chances and Life-Styles,* Glasgow: Fontana Press.

Renshaw, J., Hampson, R., Thomason, C., Darton, R., Judge, K. and Knapp, M. (1988), *Care in the Community: The First Steps,* Aldershot: Gower.

Richardson, A., Jackson, C. and Sykes,W. (1990), *Taking Research Seriously: Means of Improving and Assessing the Use and Dissemination of Research,* London: HMSO.

Richman, J.M., Rosenfeld, L.B. and Hardy, C.J. (1993), 'The Social Support Survey: A Validation Study of a Clinical Measure of the Social Support Process', *Research on Social Work Practice,* 3, 3, July 1993, Special Issue: Empirical Advances in Social Work Assessment, Sage Periodicals Press.

Rioux, M. and Bach, M. (1994), *Disability is Not Measles: New Research Paradigms in Disability*, North York, Ontario: Roeher.

Ritchie, J., Dick, D. and Lingham, R. (1994), *The Report of the Inquiry into the Care and Treatment of Christopher Clunis*, London: HMSO.
Robb, B. (1967), *Sans Everything: A Case to Answer*, London: Nelson.
Roberts, N. (1967), *Mental Health and Mental Illness,* London and New York: Routledge, Kegan Paul, the Humanities Press.
Rook, K.S. (1992), 'Detrimental Aspects of Social Relationships: Taking Stock of an Emerging Literature', in Veiel, H. and Baumann, V. (eds), *The Meaning and Measurement of Social Support,* New York: Hemisphere.
Rook, K.S. (1990), 'Parallels in the Study of Social Support and Social Strains', *Journal of Social and Clinical Psychology,* 9, 1, 118-32.
Rook, K.S. (1984), 'The Negative Side of Social Interaction: Imputation Psychological Well-being', *J. Pers. Soc. Psychology,* 46, 5, 1097-1108.
Rosenhan, D. (1973), 'On being Sane in Insane Places', *Science*, 179, 250-258.
Rosser, C. and Harris, C. (1965), *The Family and Social Change. A Study of Family and Kinship in a South Wales Town,* London: Routledge and Kegan Paul.
Salokangas, R., Palo-Oja, T. and Ojanen, M. (1991), 'The Need for Social Support Among Outpatients Suffering from Functional Psychosis', *Psychological Medicine*, 21, 209-217.
Samter, W. (1994), 'Unsupportive Relationhsips: Deficiencies in the Support-Giving Skills of the Lonely Person's Friends, in Burleson, B.R., Albrecht, T.L. and Sarason, F.G. (eds), *Communication of Social Support. Messages, Interactions, Relationships, and Community*, Ca: Sage.
Sarason, I.G., Levine, H.M., Basham, R.B. and Sarason, B.R. (1983), 'Assessing Social Support: The Social Support Questionnaire', *Journal of Personality and Social Psychology*, 44, 1, 127-139.
Sarason, I.G., Sarason, B.R. and Pierce, G.R. (1994), 'Relationship - Specific Social Support. Toward a Model for the Analysis of Supportive Interactions', in Burleson, B.R., Albrecht, T.L. and Sarason, I.G. (eds), *Communication of Social Support. Messages, Interactions, Relationships, and Community*, 91-112, Ca: Sage.
Scase, R. and Goffee, R. (1982), *The Entrepreneurial Middle Class,* London: Croom Helm.
Scull, A.T. (1984), *Decarceration: Community Treatment and the Deviant. A Radical View*, Cambridge Press (2nd edition).
Segal, S.P. and Aviram, U. (1978), *The Mentally Ill in Community-Based Sheltered Care,* New York: John Wiley and Sons.
Segal, S.P. and Holschuh, J. (1991), 'Effects of Sheltered Care Environments and Resident Characteristics on the Development of Social Networks', *Hospital and Community Psychiatry,* 42, 11, 1125-1131.
Seidel, J.V. and Clark, J.A. (1984), 'The Ethnograph: A Computer Program for the Analysis of Qualitative Data', *Qualitative Sociology*, 711-721.
Shadish, Jr. W.R. and Bootzin, R.R. (1984), 'The Social Integration of Psychiatric Patients in Nursing Homes,' *The American Journal of Psychiatry,* 141,10, 1203-1207.

Shanas, E. (1979), 'The Family as a Social Support System in Old Age', *The Gerontologist*, 19, 2, 169-174.
Shepherd, G. (1984), *Institutional Care and Rehabilitation,* Longman: London.
Silberfeld, M. (1978), 'Psychological Symptoms and Social Supports', *Social Psychiatry*, 13, 11-17.
Simic, P. (1994), 'Moving Out of Hospital into the Community', in Titterton, M. (ed.), *Caring for People in the Community: The New Welfare,* 55-76, London: J.Kingsley.
Smelser, N. J. (1963), *Theory of Collective Behaviour,* New York: Free Press.
Smith, H.W. (1975), *Strategies of Social Research: The Methodological Imagination,* London: Prentice-Hall.
Smith, A.G. and Robbins, A.E. (1982), 'Structural Ethnography: The Study of Parental Involvement', *American Behavioural Scientist*, 26, 1, 45-61.
Smith, G. and Cantley, C. (1985), *Assessing Health Care: A Study in Organisational Evaluation,* Milton Keynes: Open University.
Smith, H.L. and Thrasher, J. (1968), 'Roles, Cliques and Sanctions: Dimensions of Patient Society', in Spitzer, S.P. and Denzin, N.K. (1968), *The Mental Patient: Studies in the Sociology of Deviance,* 316-324, New York: McGraw-Hill.
Sokolovsky, J. and Cohen, C.I. (1981), 'Toward a Resolution of Methodological Dilemmas in Network Mapping', *Schizophrenia Bulletin*, 7, 1, 109-116.
Sokolovsky, J., Cohen, C.I., Berger, D. and Geiger, J. (1978), 'Personal Networks of Ex-Mental Patients in a Manhattan SRO Hotel', *Human Organisation,* 37, 1, 5-15.
Solomon, P. and Marcenko, M. (1992), 'Families of Adults with Severe Mental Illness: Their Satisfaction with Inpatient and Outpatient Treatment', *Psychosocial Rehabilitation Journal*, 16(1), 121-134,
Spicker, P., Anderson, I., Freeman, R. and McGilp, R. (1995), 'Pathways through Psychiatric Care: The Experience of Psychiatric Patients', *Health and Social Care in the Community*, 3, 6, 343-352.
Spradley, J.P. (1980), *Participant Observation,* New York: Holt, Rinehart and Winston.
Spradley, J.P. (1979), *The Ethnographic Interview,* New York: Holt, Rinehart and Winston.
Srole, L., Langner, T.S., Michael, S.T., Kirkpatrick, P., Opler, M.K. and Rennie, T.A.C. (1962), *Mental Health in the Metropolis: The Midtown Manhattan Study,* New York: McGraw-Hill.
Stein, L.I. and Test, M.A. (1980), 'Alternative to Mental Hospital Treatment, I, Conceptual Model, Treatment Program, Clinical Evaluation', *Archives of General Psychiatry*, 37, 4, 392-397.
Stombler, M. and Martin, P.Y. (1994), 'Bringing Women in, Keeping Women Down: Fratenity "Little Sister" Organisations', *Journal of Contemporary Ethnography*, 23, 150-184.
Strauss, J.S. and Carpenter, W.T. (1972), 'The Prediction of Outcome in Schizophrenia', *Archives of General Psychiatry,* 27, 739-46.

Streeter, C.L. and Franklin, C. (1992), 'Defining and Measuring Social Support: Guidelines for Social Work Practitioners', *Research on Social Work Practice*, 2, 1, January, 81-98.

Sturt, E. and Wykes, T. (1986), 'The Measurement of Social Behaviour in Psychiatric Patients: an Assessment of the Reliability and Validity of the SBS schedule', *British Journal of Psychaitry*, 148, 1-11.

Surtees, P.G. (1980), 'Social Support, Residual Adversity, and Depressive Outcome', *Social Psychiatry,* 15, 71-80.

Szasz, T.S. (ed.) (1973), *The Age of Madness: a History of Involuntary Hospitalisation,* London: Routledge and Kegan Paul.

Szasz, T.S. (1971), *The Manufacture of Madness: A Comparative Study of the Inquisition and the Mental Health Movement,* London: Routledge and Kegan Paul.

Szasz, T.S. (1961), *The Myth of Mental Illness: Foundations of a Theory of Personal Conduct*, New York: Dell.

Tardy, C.H. (1985), 'Social Support Measurement', *American Journal of Community Psychology,* 13, 187-202.

Taylor, J. and Taylor, D. (1989), *Mental Health in the 1990s: From Custody to Care?,* London: Office of Health Economics.

Taylor, R. (1994/5), 'Alienation and Integration in Mental Health Policy', *Critical Social Policy*, 42, Winter, 81-90.

Taylor, R.D.W., Huxley, P.J. and Johnson, D.A.W. (1984), 'The Role of Social Networks in the Maintenance of Schizophrenic Patients', *British Journal of Social Work,* 14, 129-140.

Team for the Assessment of Psychiatric Services (TAPS) (1990), *Better Out Than In?*, London: North East Thames Regional Psychiatric Services Health Authority.

Thornicroft, G. and Breakey, W.R. (1991), 'The COSTAR Programme. 1:Improving Social Networks of the Long-Term Mentally Ill', *British Journal of Psychiatry*, 159, 245-249.

Thornicroft, G., Gooch, C., O'Driscoll, C. and Reda, S. (1993), 'The TAPS Project 9: The Reliability of the Patient Attitude Questionnaire', *British Journal of Psychiatry*, 162 (Suppl. 19), 25-29.

Tolsdorf, C. (1976), 'Social Networks, Support and Coping: an Exploratory Study', *Family Process*, 154, 407-417.

Toomey, D.M. (1971), 'Conjugal Roles and Social Networks in an Urban Working Class Sample', *Human Relations*, 24, 5, 417-431.

Turner, S.L. (1979), 'Disability Among Schizophrenics in a Rural Community: Services and Social Support', *Research in Nursing and Health,* 2, 151-161.

Turner-Crowson, J. (1993), *Re-shaping Mental Health Services. Implications for Britain of US Experience*, Kings Fund Institute.

Twigg, J. and Atkin, K. (1994), *Carers Perceived: Policy and Practice in Informal Care*, Bukingham: Open University Press.

Uehara, E.S. (1995), 'Reciprocity Reconsidered: Gouldner's "Moral Norm of Reciprocity" and Social Support', *Journal of Social and Personal Relationships*, 12, 4, 483-502.
Unger, D.G. and Powell, D.R. (1980), 'Supporting Families Under Stress: The Role of Social Networks', *Family Relations*, 29, 566-74.
Utena, H. (1978), 'A Japanese Experience in Psychiatric Rehabilitation', *Folia Psychiatrica et Neurologica Japanica,* 32, 2, 185-189.
Vaughn, C.E. and Leff, J.P. (1976), 'The Influence of Family and Social Factors on the Course of Psychiatric Illness', *British Journal of Psychiatry*, 125, 129.
Vaux, A. (1988), *Social Support: Theory, Research and Intervention,* New York: Praeger.
Veiel, H., Crisand, M., Stroszeck-Somscher, H. and Herrie, J. (1991), 'Social Support Networks of Chronically Strained Couples: Similarity and Overlap', *Journal of Social and Personal Relationships*, 8, 279-292.
Vitalo, R. (1971), 'Teaching Improved Interpersonal Functioning as Preferred Mode of Treatment', *Journal of Clinical Psychology*, 27, 166-171.
Walker, A. (ed.) (1982), *Community Care: the Family, the State and Social Policy,* Oxford: Blackwell.
Walker, K.N., MacBride, A. and Vachon, M.L.S. (1977), 'Social Support Networks and the Crisis of Bereavement', *Social Science and Medicine*, 11, 35-41.
Walker, R. (1981), 'On the Uses of Fiction in Educational Research', in Smetherham, D. (ed.), *Practising Evaluation,* Driffield: Nafferton.
Wallace, C.J. (1984), 'Community and Interpersonal Functioning in the Course of Schizophrenic Disorders', *Schizophrenia Bulletin,* 10, 233-257.
Wallman, S. (1979), *The Scope for Ethnicity. Ethnicity at Work*, 1-14, Social Science Research Council 1979, London: MacMillan.
Warner, R.J. (1985), *Recovery From Schizophrenia,* London: Routledge and Kegan Paul.
Wax. R.H. (1971), *Doing Fieldwork. Warnings and Advice,* Chicago: University of Chicago Press.
Wayslenki, D.A., Goering, P.N., Lemire, D., Lindsey, S. and Lancee, W. (1993), 'The Hostel Outreach Program: Assertive Case Management for Homeless Mentally Ill Persons', *Hospital and Community Psychiatry*, 44, 9, 848-853.
Weber, M. (1958), *The Protestant Ethic and the Spirit of Capitalism*, New York: Charles Scribner's Sons.
Weiss, R.S. (1974), 'The Provisions of Social Relationships, in Rubin, Z. (ed.) *Doing Unto Others*, 17-26, London: Prentice-Hall.
Wellman, B. (1985), 'From Social Support to Social Network', in Sarason, I.G. and Sarason, B.R. (eds), *Social Support: Theory, Research and Applications*, 205-222, Boston: Martinus Nijhoff.
Wellman, B. (1981), 'Applying Network Analysis to the Study of Support', in Gottlieb, B.H. (ed.), *Social Networks and Social Support,* 171-200, Beverly Hills: Sage.

Welsh Office (1993), *Protocol for Investment in Health Gain: Mental Health,* Cardiff: Welsh Health Planning Forum.

Welsh Office (1989), *Mental Illness Services: A Strategy for Wales,* Cardiff: Welsh Office.

Wenger, G.C. (1994), *Understanding Support Networks and Community Care, Network Assessment for Elderly People,* Aldershot: Avebury.

Wenger, G.C. (1992), *Help in Old Age: Facing Up to Change - A Longitudinal Network Study,* Liverpool: Institute of Human Ageing, Liverpool University Press.

Wenger, G.C. (1987), *Support Networks: Change and Stability. Second Report of a Follow-up Study of Old Elderly People in North Wales,* UCW Bangor: CSPRD.

Wenger, G.C. (1984), *The Supportive Network: Coping with Old Age,* London: Allen and Unwin.

Wenger, G.C., Shahtahmasesbi, S. and Davies, R. (1991), *Morale in Old Age. Constructing and Model of Correlates of Morale,* UCW Bangor: CSPRD.

Westermeyer, J. and Pattison, E.M. (1981), 'Social Networks and Mental Illness in a Peasant Society', *Schizophrenia Bulletin,* 7, 125-134.

Williams, B. (1995), 'Users' Views of Community Mental Health Care', in Crosby, C. and Barry, M. (eds), *Community Care: Evaluation of the Provision of Mental Health Services,* Aldershot: Avebury.

Willis, J. (1989), *Drug Use and Abuse* (Popular Medicine), London: Faber and Faber.

Willmott, P. (1987), *Friendship Networks and Social Support,* London: Policy Studies Institute.

Willmott, P. and Young, M. (1962), *Family and Kinship in East London,* Harmondsworth: Penguin.

Wing, J.K. and Brown, G.W. (1970), *Institutionalisation and Schizophrenia: A Comparative Study of Three Mental Hospitals 1970-1980,* London: Cambridge University Press.

Wirth, L. (1938), 'Urbanism as a Way of Life' in Hatt, P.K. and Reiss, A.J. (eds) (1951), *Cities and Society,* 46-63, New York: Free Press.

Wolfensberger, W. (1983), 'Social Role Valorization: A Proposed New Term for the Principle of Normalisation', *Mental Retardation,* 21, 6, 235-239.

Wolfensberger, W. (1972), *Normalisation*, Canada: Canadian Institute for the Mentally Retarded.

Wong, S.E., Massel, H.K., Mark, M.D. and Liberman, R.P. (1986), 'Behaviourial Approaches to the Treatment of Schizophrenia', in Burrows, D., Norman, T.R. and Rubenstien, G. (eds), *Handbook of Studies on Schizophrenia*, 79-99, Amsterdam: Elsevier Science Publishers.

Wykes, T. (1982), 'A Hostel-Ward for "New" Long-Stay Patients: an Evaluative Study of "A Ward in a House" in Long-Term Community Care: Experience in a London Borough' (ed. J.K. Wing), 57-97, *Psychological Medicine Monograph Supplement 2.*

Wykes, T., Sturt, E. and Katz, R. (1990), 'The Prediction of Rehabilitative Success After Three Years. The Use of Social Symptom and Cognitive Variables', *British Journal of Psychiatry,* 145, 865-870.
Youll, P.J. and McCourt-Perring, C. (1993), *Raising Voices. Ensuring Quality in Residential Care*, Caring in Homes Initiative, London: HMSO.

APPENDIX 1

Hospital-Hostel Practices Profile

Restrictions on activity

1. Outside doors locked during the day
2. Restricted visiting times
3. Visits to the pub not allowed
4. Not out alone in the evening
5. Not out alone in day
6. Check that residents are in at night
7. No TV after 11 p.m.
8. Front door locked at night
9. In bed by a given time
10. Check that residents are in bed
11. Up by given time (weekday)
12. Up in mornings (weekday)
13. In by 10 p.m.
14. Encouraged to be in bed by 11 p.m.
15. Up by given time (weekend)
16. Up in the morning (weekend)
17. Movements known at weekends
18. In by given time (weekends)
19. Must stay out during day (week)
20. Set activities outside residence
21. Set domestic activities for residents
22. Not allowed razors, knives, scissors
23. Not allowed matches, lighters
24. Medicines handed out
25. Not allowed personal money
26. Belongings catalogued
27. Checked for forbidden items (admission)
28. Check for forbidden items (periodically)
29. Cannot lock own things
30. Restrictions on display of items

Meals

31. Not involved in planning meals
32. Beer not allowed
33. Spirits not allowed
34. Cannot make tea
35. Cannot make a snack
36. Set meal times

Health and hygiene

37. Weighed on admission
38. Weighed periodically
39. Dress supervised
40. No lock on toilet door
41. No lock on bathroom door
42. No choice of bathtime
43. Bathing supervised
44. Cannot wash own clothes

Residents' rooms

45. Cannot rest on bed during day
46. Staff can enter rooms
47. Opposite sex not allowed at any time
48. Cannot smoke in rooms
49. Beds made by staff

Services

50. Must ask staff for GP
51. Psychiatrist visits routinely
52. Hairdresser visits routinely
53. There are no patient-staff meetings

Index